Micrometastasis

Cancer Metastasis – Biology and Treatment

VOLUME 5

Titles published in this Series are:

Volume 1: Cancer Metastasis, Molecular and Cellular Mechanisms and Clinical Intervention.

Editors: Wen G. Jiang and Robert E. Mansel.
ISBN 0-7923-6395-7

Volume 2: Growth Factors and Receptors in Cancer Metastasis.

Editors: Wen G. Jiang, Kunio Matsumoto, and Toshikazu Nakamura.
ISBN 0-7923-7141-0

Volume 3: Cancer Metastasis – Related Genes.

Editor: Danny R. Welch
ISBN 1-4020-0522-9

Volume 4: Proteases and Their Inhibitors in Cancer Metastasis.

Editors: Jean-Michel Foidart and Ruth J. Muschel
ISBN 1-4020-0923-2

Micrometastasis

Edited by

Klaus Pantel
Director, Institute of Tumour Biology
University Hospital Hamburg-Eppendorf, Germany

KLUWER ACADEMIC PUBLISHERS
DORDRECHT / BOSTON / LONDON

A C.I.P. Catalogue record for this book is available from the Library of Congress.

ISBN 1-4020-1155-5

Published by Kluwer Academic Publishers,
P.O. Box 17, 3300 AA Dordrecht, The Netherlands.

Sold and distributed in North, Central and South America
by Kluwer Academic Publishers,
101 Philip Drive, Norwell, MA 02061, U.S.A.

In all other countries, sold and distributed
by Kluwer Academic Publishers,
P.O. Box 322, 3300 AH Dordrecht, The Netherlands.

Printed on acid-free paper

Printed in Great Britain by MPG Books Limited, Bodmin, Cornwall.

TABLE OF CONTENTS

PREFACE

Distant metastases are the main cause of cancer-related death. The onset of the metastatic process can now be assessed in cancer patients by the use of sensitive immunocytochemical and molecular methods that allow the identification of single disseminated carcinoma cells or small tumor cell clusters in regional lymph nodes, peripheral blood or distant organs.

The current assays for detection of micrometastatic tumor cells may be used to improve tumor staging with potential consequences also for subsequent adjuvant therapy. Another promising clinical application is monitoring the response of micrometastatic cells in blood and bone marrow to adjuvant therapies, which, at present, can only be assessed retrospectively after an extended period of clinical follow-up. Moreover, tools recently established in several laboratories allow us to obtain further insights into the phenotype and genotype of micrometastases. Identification of the molecular determinants of micrometastatic cells may help to design new strategies to detect and eliminate minimal residual cancer.

In this book, leading experts in the area of micrometastasis research provide an overview that summarizes the current state of research on micrometastatic disease in patients with solid tumors. In each chapter, the technical aspect as well as clinical relevance of micrometastasis detection is discussed.

I hope the knowledge provided in this book will help the reader to understand the importance of this rather new field of clinical cancer research.

Professor Dr. Klaus Pantel
Editor

LIST OF CONTRIBUTORS

Ruud H. Brakenhoff. *Section Tumour Biology, Department of Otolaryngology/ Head-Neck Surgery, Vrije Universiteit Medical Center*

Stephan Braun. *Universitätsklinik für Frauenheilkunde, Leopold-Franzens-Univerrsität, Anichstrasse 35, A-6020 Innsbruck, Austria*

Richard J. Cote. *Keck School of Medicine at the University of Southern California/Kenneth Norris Comprehensive Cancer Center, Los Angeles, California, USA*

William J. Ellis. *Department of Urology, University of Washington Medical School, Seattle, USA*

Petra Goldin-Lang. *Department of Medicine III, University Hospital Benjamin Franklin, Free University Berlin, Hindenburgdamm 30, 12200 Berlin, Germany*

Debra Hawes. *Keck School of Medicine at the University of Southern California/Kenneth Norris Comprehensive Cancer Center, Los Angeles, California, USA*

Stefan B. Hosch. *Department of General and Thoracic Surgery, Universitätsklinikum Eppendorf, Martinistrasse 52, D-20246 Hamburg, Germany*

Jacob R. Izbicki. *Department of General and Thoracic Surgery, Universitätsklinikum Eppendorf, Martinistrasse 52, D-20246 Hamburg, Germany*

Holger Kalthoff. *Molecular Oncology Research Group, Department for General and Thoracic Surgery, University Hospital of Schleswig-Holstein, Campus Kiel, Germany*

Ulrich Keilholz. *Department of Medicine III, University Hospital Benjamin Franklin, Free University Berlin, Hindenburgdamm 30, 12200 Berlin, Germany*

William H. Krüger. *Internal Medicine C - Haematology/Oncology, Ernst-Moritz-Arndt-University, Greifswald, Germany*

Paul H. Lange. *Department of Urology, University of Washington Medical School, Seattle, USA*

Volkmar Müller. *Institut für Tumorbiologie, Klinik für Frauenheilkunde, Universitätsklinikum Eppendorf, Martinistrasse 52, D-20246 Hamburg, Germany*

A. Munro Neville. *Ludwig Institute for Cancer Research, London, UK*

Klaus Pantel. *Institut für Tumorbiologie, Universitätsklinikum Eppendorf, Martinistrasse 52, D-20246 Hamburg, Germany*

Bernward Passlick. *Department of Surgery, Division of Thoracic Surgery, University of Munich, Germany*

Jesco Pfitzenmaier. *Department of Urology, University of Washington Medical School, Seattle, USA*

Peter Scheuemann. *Department of General and Thoracic Surgery, Universitätsklinikum Eppendorf, Martinistrasse 52, D-20246 Hamburg, Germany*

Robert L. Vessella. *Department of Urology, University of Washington Medical School, Seattle, USA*

Ilka Vogel. *Molecular Oncology Research Group, Department for General and Thoracic Surgery, University Hospital of Schleswig-Holstein, Campus Kiel, Germany*

Chapter 1

TECHNICAL ASPECTS OF THE DETECTION OF DISSEMINATED TUMOUR CELLS BY MOLECULAR METHODS

William H. Krüger

Internal Medicine C - Haematology/Oncology, Ernst-Moritz-Arndt-University, Greifswald, Germany

Abstract

The standard method for the detection of disseminated epithelial tumour cells is still immunocytochemistry despite some concerns such as relative low sensitivity and subjective evaluation. Several approaches have been made to develop sensitive and specific polymerase-chain reaction assays comparable to those in use for detection of minimal residual disease in haematological malignancies. The major problem is the absence of specific genetic aberrations in solid cancer. Thus, researchers focused on amplification of so-called tissue-specific expressed genes such as epithelial structure proteins or messenger RNA of tumour markers or tumour-associated proteins. Most assays were described as highly specific valuable tools by the developers, and subsequently as non-specific by investigators. This chapter describes the mechanisms leading to so-called 'false-positive' and 'false-negative' results, and discusses the strength and weakness of RT-PCR for detection of solid cancer cells. Furthermore, strategies are discussed for development of reverse-transcriptase polymerase-chain reaction systems and for using and increasing their specificity.

INTRODUCTION

Dissemination of solid tumours in the bone marrow or blood stream has been described for a variety of malignancies. The term 'disseminated tumour cells' or 'early tumour cell dissemination' usually means a very low amount of tumour cells in the marrow not detectable by routine microscopy of marrow or blood slides (1).

Molecular methods for the detection of minimal residual disease were first used in haematological malignancies such as non-Hodgkin's lymphoma or acute lymphocytic leukaemia (ALL) (2). Southern blot analysis detecting B-cell or T-cell specific rearrangements or genetic aberrations had a relative poor sensitivity between 1% and 5% (3, 4). The milestone was the description of the

K. Pantel (ed.), Micrometastasis, 1–18.

polymerase-chain reaction (PCR) technique for *in vitro* gene amplification in the mid-1980s. This technique allows a nearly exponential multiplication of a DNA-fragment with a pair of specific nucleotides called primers using a repetitive temperature profile for denaturation, primer-annealing and polymerization of DNA (5). The PCR-technique can be used for the sensitive detection of DNA-fragments, as well as for the detection of mRNA-templates after transcription into a cDNA in a reverse-transcriptase reaction (6).

Some haematological neoplasms bear optimal aberrations for PCR detection of minimal residual disease. The translocation T(14;18) is common in follicular lymphoma and can be amplified from DNA without reverse transcription. The second classic chromosomal aberration is the so-called Philadelphia-chromosome T(9;22) or bcr/abl-rearrangement in chronic myeloid leukaemia (CML). The molecular detection of T(9;22) requires necessarily transcription of mRNA into cDNA due to the varying size of the corresponding chromosomal DNA-segment. Both assays have been used with great success for the detection of minimal residual disease (6, 7). A positive signal in bcr/abl-PCR has become an indication for treatment of early relapse of CML after allogeneic stem cell transplantation by donor-lymphocyte infusions (8).

METHODS FOR THE DETECTION OF DISSEMINATED TUMOUR CELLS

The standard method for the detection of disseminated epithelial cancer is the immunocytochemical staining of epithelial-specific gene products commonly not expressed in haemopoietic cells such as cytokeratins or mucins (1). The sensitivity of this technique depends on the amount of cells examined and was initially quite poor due to the fact that most groups investigated not more than 2×10^5 mononucleated cells. This standard was increased to a minimum of 2×10^6 during the last years; however, RT PCR offers sensitivity up to $1/10^7$ and its evaluation is nearly independent from investigator's bias (9).

In contrast to haematological malignancies specific chromosomal aberrations useful for detection of minimal disease by PCR-technique cannot regularly be found in epithelial tumour cells (10). The basic consideration in development of PCR assays for the specific detection of solid cancer cells in blood, bone marrow or peripheral stem cell aphereses was that epithel-derived cells do not usually occur in haemopoietic compartments. Thus, the development of PCR-techniques focused on the amplification of so-called lineage-specific transcribed genes obviously not expressed in haemopoietic cells (9). Knowledge from immunohistochemical tumour cell detection was transferred upstream to the mRNA-level. The easy upstream transfer carries a couple of pitfalls and may lead to 'false-positive' or 'false-negative' results of PCR assays. However, here it must be pointed out that in this text 'false-positive' or 'false-negative' means specific and correct results, but false in relation to the presence or absence of tumour cells in the sample. The pitfalls of the PCR-reaction itself will not be discussed in this chapter. Furthermore, not all gene sequences employed for cancer cell detection will be discussed here, rather the mechanisms leading to 'false-positive' or 'false-negative' results will be elucidated.

TARGET SEQUENCES FOR MOLECULAR DETECTION OF DISSEMINATED SOLID CANCER CELLS

Carcinoembryonic Antigen (CEA)

The carcinoembryonic antigen has long been in use as the classic serological tumour marker of large bowel cancer (11). Cancer cells of gastrointestinal origin preferably secrete the protein; however, mRNA usually can likewise be detected in breast cancer cells. Gerhard *et al.* have developed a two-step nested PCR for the detection of cancer cells in cells of haemopoietic origin with a sensitivity of 5×10^6. 56 samples obtained from healthy volunteers or patients without epithelial malignancies scored negative, whereas the CEA-message could be detected in 14 of 21 specimens from patients with gastrointestinal cancer or breast cancer (12). Subsequently, the CEA-RT-PCR was used by two Japanese groups with success for the detection of occult cancer cells in lymph nodes (13, 14).

Cytokeratins

Cytokeratins are structure-proteins ubiquitously expressed by epithelial cells. Pathologists use the immunohistochemical detection of cytokeratins in cells of unknown origin to prove their epithelial derivation. A variety of different cytokeratins have been described. For most of them so-called pseudogenes exist. These pseudogenes are sections of genomic DNA whose base sequence is identical to that of the spliced mRNA (15). PCR assays for the detection of disseminated epithelial cancer have been developed amplifying RNA-sequences of the cytokeratins 18, 19 and 20 (16–18). Datta and Fields detected with their CK19-RT-PCR assays disseminated breast cancer cells in blood, bone marrow and peripheral stem cell collections (19, 20). Other groups used the CK19 reverse transcriptase polymerase-chain reaction for the detection of disseminated gastrointestinal cancer cells or for analysis of lymph nodes (21, 22). An assay amplifying the sequence of the cytokeratin-20 message has been used successfully for the detection of circulating cells of gastrointestinal cancer (23). However, here it must be mentioned that the cytokeratin-20 protein is commonly expressed by gastrointestinal cancer but not by breast cancer cells (24).

Hormonal Receptor Genes

An assay amplifying the sequence of the epithelial growth factor receptor (EGF-R) was used by one group to monitor an immunomagnetical approach to purge stem cell apheresis samples from contaminating breast cancer cells in an *in vitro* system. Further data concerning this assay are not published (25).

Mucins and Breast-associated Antigens

Mucins are highly glycosylated proteins located in the membrane of epithelial cells (26). These epitopes were used by various investigators for the immunological detection of occult epithelial cancer cells (27, 28). Immunological cross reactions with cells of the haemopoietic systems have been described by various groups using different techniques such as immunocytochemistry and FACS analysis (29–31).

Noguchi *et al.* published a sensitive and specific RT-PCR assay amplifying the MUC1 message for the detection of breast cancer cells in lymph nodes. The results were superior to those obtained by conventional immunocytochemistry (32). However, these positive experiences with MUC1-RT-PCR could not be reproduced by other investigators.

Mammaglobin is a protein from the family of the uteroglobins genetically located on chromosome 11q13. The protein can be found in human tear fluid, in breast epithel cells and overexpressed in malignant breast tissue (33, 34). A couple of RT-PCR assays for the detection of occult breast cancer cells have been published. Zach *et al.* investigated 114 peripheral blood samples from 68 women with breast cancer. A total of 29 (25%) of these specimens scored positive, whereas the message could not be amplified from 27 samples from healthy volunteers (35).

Proteins of the human milk fat complex were used by several investigators as targets for the immunological cancer cell detection (36). The group of Larocca and Ceriani cloned and sequenced two proteins named breast-associated antigens BA46 and BA70. Immunological studies suggested that these epitopes could be feasible targets for immunotherapeutic approaches of breast cancer treatment, and sequence analysis excluded homologies to other mucin genes (37, 38). The results of the evaluation of the breast-associated antigens BA46 and BA70 for the molecular detection of breast cancer cells are discussed below.

A variety of RT-PCR assays amplifying different target sequences have been described as sensitive and specific tools for the detection of disseminated breast cancer cells by their developers. However, the promising results could mostly not be reproduced by subsequent investigators. The mechanisms leading to these so-called 'false-positive' results had not been investigated so far and RT-PCR often was prejudiced as general non-specific for the detection of epithelial cancer cells.

MECHANISMS LEADING TO FALSE-NEGATIVE OR FALSE-POSITIVE RESULTS

Preanalytical Considerations

Amplification of Pseudogene Sequences

Pseudogenes are non-transcribed genomic DNA-sequences identical or very similar to the messenger-RNA derived from the original gene. Pseudogenes are described for a variety of genes including often as positive-control in RT-PCR assays using β-actin mRNA and the majority of cytokeratins. The exclusion of an accidental pseudogene amplification in RT-PCR assays is mandatory prior to its use for tumour cell detection (16). For discrimination of mRNA- and DNA-derived amplicons obtained by an RT-PCR assay each primer pair must span at least one intron, as shown in Figure 1. Then amplicons derived from genomic DNA and from mRNA can be discriminated by their different size. DNA-derived fragments are always larger than those derived from mRNA (Figure 2). However, by this practical approach it may not always be possible to discriminate between

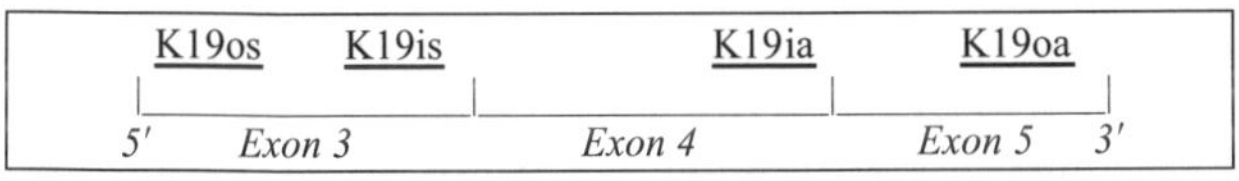

Figure 1. Genomic localization of primers used for amplification of the cytokeratin-19 message. Each primer pair spans at least one intron.

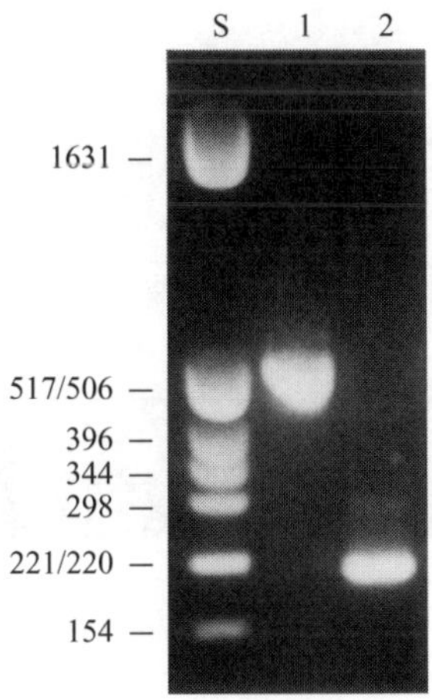

Figure 2. Amplifiction of genomic DNA (1) and messenger-RNA after reverse transcription (2) with cytokeratin-19 RT-PCR; S: standard in base pairs.

an accidental pseudogene amplification and an incorrect choice of primers without span of at least one intron (17).

Transcription Varies among Distinct Epithelial Target Cell Populations

Among the cytokeratins there are some such as cytokeratin-18 or cytokeratin-19 ubiquitously expressed in epithelial cancer cells. The related gene products serve as general targets for the immunological detection and identification of epithelial cells in haemopoietic compartments (15). Cytokeratin-20 has been described as a useful target sequence for molecular detection of disseminated gastrointestinal cancer cells (23). A major advantage compared to other cytokeratins is the obvious lack of related pseudogene-sequences. However, for breast cancer the situation is completely different. Neither revealed immunological studies any evidence for the expression of cytokeratin-20 by breast cancer cells nor could any strong signals be amplified from breast cancer cell lines (39).

Strong Constitutional Transcription and Protein Synthesis in Haemopoietic Cells

The good experiences with a MUC-1 RT-PCR for detection of occult epithelial cancer cells published by a group from Japan has not been duplicated by other groups so far. The MUC-1 sequences could be amplified from varying haemopoietic cell lines of lymphoid and myeloid origin. Furthermore, the strong signal was obtained when mRNA from bone marrow from healthy volunteer donors was subjected to amplification. Both groups have used independent RT-PCR assays with different primer pairs. These results clearly showed that the

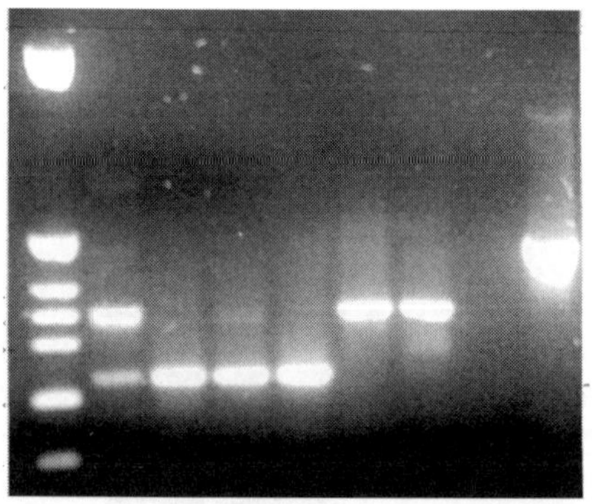

Figure 3. PCR-amplification of MUC1-mRNA after reverse transcription. Lane 1: pBR322/Hinf-III (1640/516/507/396/344/298/220/221/194 base pairs); lane 2: Raji; lane 3: K562; lane 4: bone marrow; lane 5: MCF7 (all mRNA-derived); lane 6: Raji; lane 7: MCF7 (both genomic DNA); lane 8: H_2O; lane 9: positive control (Perkin-Elmer).

MUC1 message is constitutionally transcribed by haemopoietic cells and that this phenomenon is not related to a gene deregulation in malignant cells only (Figure 3) (40, 41).

These results did not absolutely surprise due to the fact that expression of mucin epitopes by haemopoietic cells has been published by at least three groups (29–31). However, it must be mentioned that antibodies against mucin epitopes could be useful for identification of disseminated epithelial cancer cells despite these disappointing results on the molecular level. Mucins are highly glycosylated molecules whose antigeneity might become modified by glycosylation. There are some hints that mucins might be functionally expressed in haemopoietic cells but little research has been done in this field so far.

The expression of mucin-related proteins in haemopoietic cells was analysed for the mammary epithelium-related antigens BA46 (lactadherin) and BA70 in lymphoid and myeloid cell lines, and in clinical specimens. By Northern-hybridization with specific oligonucleotides a ubiquitous transcription of both genes, independent from the provenance of cells or the chromosomal gender, was found. Both mRNA molecules were amplified by RT-PCR from the samples and the specificity could be confirmed by sequence analysis. Peptide-specific antibodies were raised in rabbits and used for Western-blot analysis and for immunocytochemical studies. Both antibodies reacted with total cell lysates from myeloid and lymphatic cells. In immunocytochemistry antibody P717 (anti BA46, anti-lactadherin) had a significant strong staining of the myeloid cell lines K562 and HL60 suggesting a participation of lactadherin in leukocyte-function. Using antibody P718 (anti BA70), strong stains were seen in myeloid line K562 and lymphoid line ST486 (Figure 4). In conclusion, these findings expanded the results that the concept of lineage-specific gene expression is no longer valid at the molecular level (42).

Induction of Transcription by Cytokines *in vitro* and *in vivo*

The first evidence for a possible induction of cytokeratin-19 message in cells related to the haemopoietic system under certain conditions was a publication by Traweek in 1993 (43). The cytokeratin-19 message was amplified from cultured fibroblasts and endothelial cells but neither from normal lymphatic tissue nor from bone marrow. It can be assumed that these haemopoietic specimens always contain a distinct number of endothelial cells and fibroblasts.

The induction of epithelium-related genes in haemopoietic cells under *in vivo* and *in vitro* conditions has been clearly shown for the cytokeratin-19 and carcinoembryonic antigen messages. Bone marrow, granulocyte colony-stimulating factor (G-CSF)-mobilized blood stem cells and peripheral blood samples obtained from healthy volunteers ($n = 15$; CEA $n = 7$), from patients with epithelial ($n = 29$) and haematological ($n = 23$) cancer and from patients with chronic inflammatory diseases ($n = 16$) were examined for the transcription of CEA and CK19. Neither CEA nor cytokeratin-19 messages could be amplified

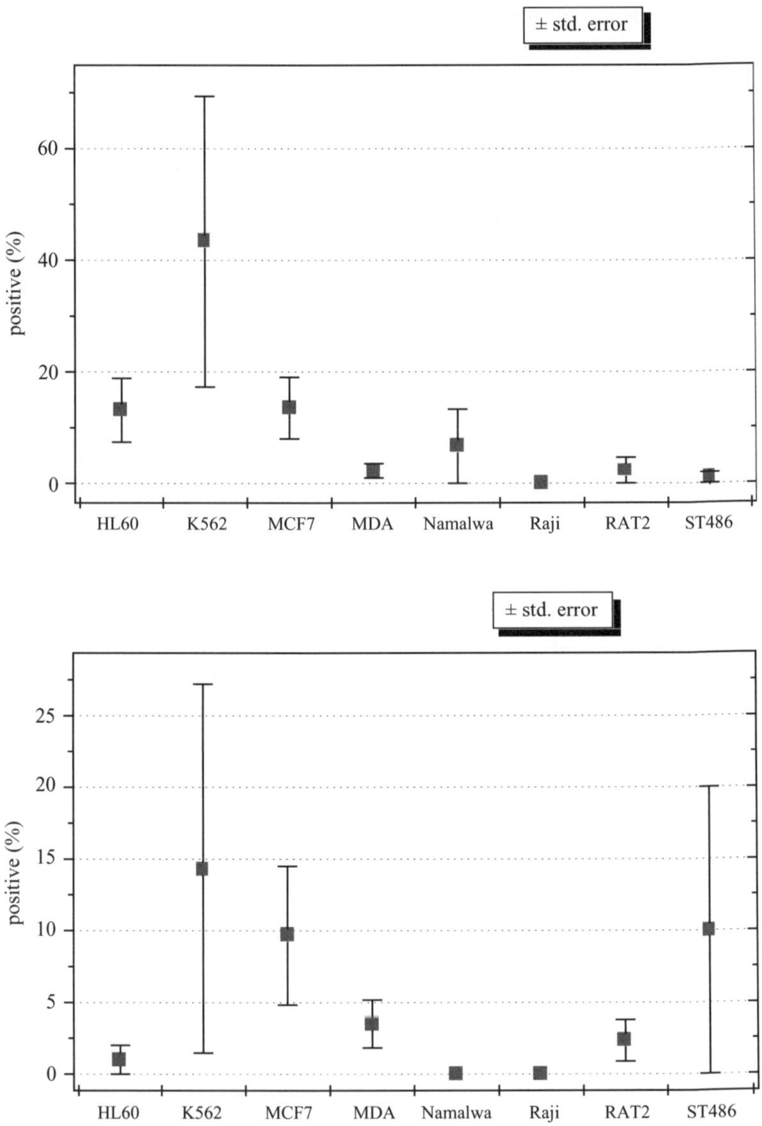

Figure 4. Labelling of cells with polyclonal antibodies against BA46 (lactadherin) (top) and BA70 (bottom). Shown is the percentage of stained cells by immunocytochemistry performed on cytospin slides (MDA: MDA-MB453).

from bone marrow samples from healthy subjects and from patients with haematological malignancies. In contrast, specimens from patients with inflammatory diseases such as ulcerative colitis or Crohn's disease scored positive up to 60%. To investigate the influence of inflammation on target mRNA expression, haemopoietic cells were cultured with and without cytokine stimulation *in vitro*.

CK19 messages could be easily detected in cultured marrow cells without further stimulation, CEA messages only after gamma-interferon (γ-INF) stimulation. These results are in accordance with data obtained using stimulated HT 29 cells. It is known that γ-interferon and TNF-α lead to an upregulation of the CEA message in HT 29 cells *in vitro* and that the CEA-gene contains a γ-interferon responsive element. In contrast, G-CSF-mobilized peripheral blood stem cells were positive for CK19 messages only after stem cell factor (SCF) or interleukin stimulation (Table 1). These results lead us to conclude: 1) cytokeratin-19 mRNA transcription is easily induced in bone marrow in the presence of stromal cells; 2) that under specific and very artificial conditions cytokeratin transcription is also possible in haemopoietic precursor cells extracted from peripheral blood; and 3) the detected specific cytokeratin mRNA in patients with chronic inflammatory diseases may be induced in stromal cells of the reactive marrow by cytokines involved in the inflammatory process (44).

Table 1. PCR-amplification of cytokeratin-19 and CEA messages from cultured non-stimulated and cytokine-stimulated leukocytes from healthy bone marrow (BM) and G-CSF-mobilized leukaphereses samples (LP), and peripheral blood (PB). PB was examined after three-day (d3) culture due to decreasing cell count

Sample	d1	d7	d7 (SCF)	d7 (G-CSF)	d7 (GM-CSF)	d7 (IL3)	d7 (IL6)	d7 (γINF)
CK19								
BM	–	+	+	+	+	+	+	(+)
LP	–	–	+	–	–	+/–	+/–	–
CEA								
BM	–	–	–	–	–	–	–	+
PB	–	– (d3)	n.d.	n.d.	n.d.	n.d.	n.d.	+ (d3)

Table 2. Cytokeratin-20 RT-PCR results in cell lines without and after cytokine stimulation. Shown is the number of culture experiments scoring positive in CK20-RT-PCR of all culture experiments performed; e.g., 1 of 3 means that stimulation experiment was performed in triplicate and CK20 message could be amplified from one of these cultures. All positive results are shaded

Cell line	w/o	IL3	IL6	IL1β	SCF	INFγ	FLT3	TPO	G-CSF	GM-CSF
Fibroblasts	0 of 4	0 of 2	0 of 2	0 of 2	0 of 2	0 of 2	0 of 2	0 of 2	0 of 2	0 of 2
HL60	0 of 6	0 of 3	0 of 3	0 of 3	0 of 3	0 of 3	1 of 3	0 of 3	0 of 3	0 of 3
K562	6 of 13	1 of 3	0 of 3	2 of 3	0 of 3	1 of 3	0 of 3	1 of 3	1 of 3	1 of 3
Raji	0 of 7	0 of 2	0 of 2	0 of 2	0 of 2	0 of 2	1 of 2	0 of 2	0 of 2	0 of 2
TF1	0 of 6	0 of 2	0 of 2	0 of 2	0 of 2	0 of 2	0 of 2	0 of 2	0 of 2	0 of 2
U937	0 of 8	0 of 2	0 of 2	0 of 2	0 of 2	0 of 2	0 of 2	0 of 2	0 of 2	0 of 2

The approach to investigate a possible induction of cytokeratin-20 and mammaglobin messages in haemopoietic cells was completely different (39). Bone marrow, cytokine-mobilized stem cells and blood samples were exposed to a panel of cytokines *in vitro* prior to amplification of the cytokeratin and mammaglobin messages. The detection of 12% and 7% positive results in non-stimulated native samples from patients without epithelial cancer in this study do not support prior

Table 3. Mammaglobin RT-PCR results in cell lines without and after cytokine stimulation. Shown is the number of culture experiments scoring positive in MG-RT-PCR of all culture experiments performed; e.g., 1 of 3 means that stimulation experiment was performed in triplicate and CK20 message could be amplified from one of these cultures. Partly positive results are light and completely positive results are shaded dark. Significant differences were calculated by Chi-square test and shown when appropriate

Cell line	w/o	IL3	IL6	IL1β	SCF	INFγ	FLT3	TPO	G-CSF	GM-CSF
Fibroblasts	4 of 4	2 of 2	2 of 2	2 of 2	2 of 2	2 of 2	2 of 2	2 of 2	2 of 2	2 of 2
HL60	3 of 6	0 of 3	0 of 3	2 of 3	1 of 3	0 of 3	2 of 3	1 of 3	0 of 3	2 of 3
K562	2 of 11	1 of 3	2 of 3	1 of 3	1 of 3	2 of 3	1 of 3	2 of 3	2 of 3	2 of 3
Raji	4 of 7	2 of 2	2 of 2	2 of 2	2 of 2	2 of 2	1 of 2	2 of 2	2 of 2	2 of 2
TF1	2 of 6	1 of 2	2 of 2	1 of 2	2 of 2	2 of 2	2 of 2	2 of 2	2 of 2	2 of 2
U937	5 of 10	1 of 2	1 of 2	2 of 2	1 of 2	0 of 2	2 of 2	0 of 2	0 of 2	1 of 2
pos. (%)	*45*	*50*	*64*	*71*	*64*	*57*	*71*	*64*	*57*	*79 ($p = 0.01$)*

Table 4. CK20- and MG-RT-PCR results in clinical specimens prior to culture and after culture with and without stimulation. A total of 22 samples consisting of bone marrow ($n = 11$) and leukapheresis samples ($n = 11$) was investigated. Shown is the percentage of positive results. Significant differences between non-stimulated cultures (w/o) and each stimulation-experiment were calculated by Chi-square test and shown when appropriate (39)

CYTOKINE	CK20 RT-PCR	MG RT-PCR
w/o	12	7
SCF	0	15
G-CSF	12	13
GM-CSF	0	24 $p < 0.01$
IL-3	6	24 $p < 0.01$
IL-6	22	11
γINF	8	27 $p < 0.003$
IL-1β	19	13
FLT3	5	10
TPO	15	30 $p < 10^{-3}$

reported good results for CK20- and MG-RT-PCR (Table 4). To investigate the biological base of these results, cell lines of myeloid and lymphoid lineage and fibroblasts have been examined for the transcription of both genes. Additionally, to investigate biological interference of both assays, cell lines have been stimulated by varying cytokines prior to reverse-transcriptase polymerase-chain reactions. Furthermore, the clinical samples consisting of bone marrow and leukapheresis samples obtained from patients without epithelial cancer were also cultured and exposed to different cytokines. This approach was chosen in order to bring as close as possible the *in vivo* situation with interactions between different cell populations. The results were completely different for cytokeratin-20- and mammaglobin RT-PCR. The myeloid cell line K562, derived from a blast crisis of a chronic myeloid leukaemia, scored positive in approximately one-third of the CK20-RT-PCR assays performed. No other cell line, except HL60 and Raji after additional FLT3-stimulation in one-third of experiments, scored positive for CK20 mRNA, either without or with cytokine-supplementation. The CK20-amplification from HL60-cells can be explained by their myeloid origin. However, it remains unclear for Raji (Table 2). These results support a recent study, which describes a low-level background-transcription of the CK20-gene in granulocytes as one reason for a so-called non-specific amplification in the RT-PCR assay (45). In accordance with the results obtained from cell lines, the exposition of bone marrow and leukapheresis samples to cytokines did not lead to a significant change. Percentage of positive results after stimulation varied between 0% and 22% without any evident patterns or significant differences from non-stimulated samples (Table 4). For the routine approach this interference cannot be overcome simply by removal of granulocytes by ficoll-separation due to the fact that tumour cells might be lost by this separation method (46).

All cell lines scored positive in a high percentage for the mammaglobin message. No evident differences between lymphoid and myeloid cells were seen. However, it should be pointed out that fibroblasts were positive in 100%. Surprisingly, the picture changed completely when the results from all cell lines were combined for each cytokine. The percentage of positive results increased after stimulation from 45% to 50% up to 78%. For GM-CSF the increase was significant (Table 3). The results obtained from cultured cell lines were, as seen for the CK20 amplification, confirmed by the investigation of stimulated clinical samples. All cytokines led to an increased detection rate varying from 11% to 30% (Table 4). Even here, the difference was significant for GM-CSF. Surprisingly, the strongest induction was seen after stimulation with γINF or TPO. These results cannot be explained by this study. However, it can be clearly concluded that the mammaglobin message can be induced by cytokines. Also supportive for this conclusion is the observation that without stimulation the percentage of positive results is higher for cytokeratin-20 than for mammaglobin (12% vs. 7%) due to the background transcription in granulocytes. After stimulation with different cytokines, the percentage of positive results is higher in seven out of nine experiments for mammaglobin as compared to cytokeratin-20.

These findings suggest that interactions of different cell populations can at least enhance this induction. Routine use of mammaglobin-amplification, even in real-time PCR, is handicapped by this interference due to the fact that the intensity of induction is unknown and cannot be overcome by definition of a cut-off value.

For both assays it can be concluded that biological interference might disturb the specific amplification and might lead to so-called false-positive results. The pathways of non-tumour cell-specific amplification are different for the cytokeratin-20 and mammaglobin genes as described recently for the CEA- and CK19-RT-PCR assays (44).

The presented data clearly show that transcription of so-called tissue-specific genes may be induced in haemopoietic tissues under certain conditions. Furthermore, they show that the patterns of induction are completely different for varying genes even from the same family. These differences in induction patterns demonstrate that the so-called non-specific gene expression is not only a phenomenon from a non-specific stimulation.

Analytical Considerations

Low-level Background Transcription in Distinct Cell Populations and their Removal

The stimulation experiments clearly showed that the transcription of the cytokeratin-20 message in haemopoietic cells is limited to differentiated cells of myeloid origin (Table 2) (39). It could be criticized that this observation could be only a phenomenon of gene deregulation in malignant cells. However, the thesis of a low-level background transcription was supported by a second investigation. In this study the diagnostic specificity of the CK20 mRNA detection in samples from healthy donors (HD; $n = 33$), intensive care units patients (ICU; $n = 20$) and bone marrow obtained from patients suffering from chronic inflammatory diseases (CID; $n = 14$) was investigated. RNAs purified from stabilized lysates showed positive results in 24% of the HD group (8/33), 35% of the ICU group (8/20) and in 40% of the CID group (5/14). The use of Ficoll gradients to separate nucleated cells completely restored the specificity of this CK20 RT-PCR assay. The CK20-expressing cells are positively identified to belong to the granulocyte fraction of leucocytes, which appear to express the gene on a background level (45).

A significant loss of tumour cells by Ficoll centrifugation compared to ammonium chloride mediated red cell lysis was shown recently. However, the same publication found no negative effect of centrifugation on sensitivity of tumour cell detection by molecular methods so far (46).

An overview about the genetic mechanisms leading to false-positive or false-negative results is shown in Table 5. The variety of mechanisms leading to

Table 5. Mechanisms of gene interference leading to false-positive or false-negative results in RT-PCR assays (references in the text)

Mechanism	Gene	Impact on RT-PCR
Pseudogene-amplification	CK18, CK19	False-positive
Constitutional strong transcription and protein synthesis	MUC1, BA46, BA70	False-positive
Induction by cytokines	CEA, CK19	False-positive
Background transcription enhanced by cytokines	MG	False-positive
Background transcription in distinct haemopoietic subpopulations	CK20	False-positive
Transcription only in epithelial subpopulations	CK20, MG	False-negative

a so-called 'illegitimate' gene expression lead to the conclusion that the transcription of the investigated genes in haemopoietic cells is specific and probably has any biological function and is not only a non-specific background-phenomenon as postulated by other investigators (47, 48).

STRATEGIES FOR THE DEVELOPMENT AND EVALUATION OF A REVERSE TRANSCRIPTASE PCR FOR THE DETECTION OF SOLID CANCER CELLS

A candidate gene for a new RT-PCR assay for the detection of disseminated cancer cells should principally be chosen on the base of immunohistochemical studies investigating its expression in the potential target cells. An expression by cell populations of compartment searched for cancer cells disqualifies the gene for further investigation. Sequences of candidate genes and messages should be retrieved from data bases such as ENTREZ (http://www.ncbi.nlm.nih.gov/Entrez) at NCBI or HUSAR (http://genome.dkfz-heidelberg.de) at DKFZ. Choice and design of primers must consider the intron/exon structure of the gene and sequences of eventually existent pseudogenes. A primer pair must span at least one intron as shown in Figure 1.

The primer pairs should be tested for their mRNA-specificity by amplifying cellular DNA and mRNA-derived cDNA from a positive control separately. Here the amplification of cellular DNA leads to a significant increase in size of the amplicon compared to the mRNA-derived amplicon Figure 2. Identical sizes of cellular DNA- and mRNA-derived amplification products indicate either the accidental amplification of a pseudogenes or the lack of exon/exon junctions within the amplicon and in each case the uselessness of the tested primers.

In the next step of RT-PCR-development negative bone marrow, cytokine-mobilized stem cells, peripheral vein blood, lymphatic tissues or other specimens planned to be searched for cancer cells should be examined. Furthermore, investigation of a couple of cell lines of the same tissue type as the disseminated cancer cells to be detected by RT-PCR must be tested and should give constant positive and strong results. Then the sensitivity can be determined by investigation of diluted cancer cells in nucleated blood cells. The mechanisms of so-called illegitimate transcription as discussed above must be considered prior to the investigation of clinical samples. This means, for example, when bone marrow of patients with co-existent chronic inflammatory disease shall be searched for cancer cells the assay must be validated with samples obtained from patients without cancer, but with the same co-disease, or more simply: each assay must be validated under test conditions.

CONCLUSION

Currently there is no further evidence for a general non-specificity of RT-PCR assays designed for the detection of disseminated solid cancer cells. The mechanisms leading to so-called false-positive results in PCR assays have been investigated and it has been shown that these so-called 'false-positive' results are 'true-positive' and indeed derived by specific amplification-reactions. In contrast to haematological malignancies bearing specific translocations such as T(9;22) or T(14;18), the situation for solid tumours is completely different. It is nearly impossible to exclude any low-level transcription in haemopoietic cells. However, the specific detection of tumour cells will be increased by combination of different assays using targets with different pathways to transcription in haemopoietic cells. For investigation of liquid compartments such as bone marrow or peripheral stem cells the conventional immunocytochemistry remains the standard. The limitations of tumour cell detection by RT-PCR are quite similar as those established two decades ago for serological tumour marker detection (11). It must be pointed out that RT-PCR is no feasible tool for a screening of undefined large populations for the presence of tumour cells in bone marrow or peripheral blood. Sensitivity of immunocytochemistry can be increased impressively by immunomagnetic cancer cell enrichment prior to immunocytochemistry, but even here a significant loss of tumour cells is seen due to variation in expression of antigens used for selection procedure.

To perform PCR-analysis after immunomagnetic pre-enrichment does not make sense due to the fact that the positive-enriched fraction can be easily investigated on one cytospin slide in a single or double stain immunocytochemistry (49). In conclusion, the RT-PCR-technique is a powerful tool to determine the absence of tumour cells in samples investigated with a high specificity and sensitivity. Furthermore, it will facilitate examination of lymphatic tissue samples for cancer cells such as lymph nodes, which cannot be easily spun onto cytospin slides for immunocytochemistry. A possible important field of application could be the optimization of auxiliary lymph node staging of women with newly diagnosed breast cancer or staging of mesenterial lymph nodes of patients with colorectal cancer. Comparison of RT-PCR with immunocytochemistry stands out so far. Quantitative amplification by real-time PCR has become available but there is some concern. First, it is not known if the level of target antigen transcription is constant in searched cell populations; and second it is unknown if it correlates between cell lines and disseminated tumour cells. Prior to introduction of real-time PCR into diagnosis of disseminated solid tumours the place of conventional PCR within options of diagnostic tools should be defined.

REFERENCES

1. Pantel K. Detection of minimal disease in patients with solid tumours. J Hematother. 1996; 5:359–367.
2. Radich J. Minimal residual disease. Curr Opin Hematol. 1995; 2:300–304.
3. Van Dongen JJ, Wolvers-Tettero IL. Analysis of immunoglobulin and T cell receptor genes. Part II: Possibilities and limitations in the diagnosis and management of lymphoproliferative diseases and related disorders. Clin Chim Acta. 1991; 198:93–174.
4. Van Dongen JJ, Wolvers-Tettero IL. Analysis of immunoglobulin and T cell receptor genes. Part I: Basic and technical aspects. Clin Chim Acta. 1991; 198:1–91.
5. Sambrook J, Fritsch EF, Maniatis T. Molecular Cloning. 2nd ed. Cold Spring Harbor: Laboratory Press, 1989.
6. Gribben J, Nadler L. Detection of minimal residual disease. Cancer Treat Res. 1995; 76:249–270.
7. Cross NC. Minimal residual disease in chronic myeloid leukaemia. Hematol Cell Ther. 1998; 40:224–228.
8. Baurmann H, Nagel S, Binder T, Neubauer A, Siegert W, Huhn D. Kinetics of the graft-versus-leukemia response after donor leukocyte infusions for relapsed chronic myeloid leukemia after allogeneic bone marrow transplantation. Blood. 1998; 92:3582–3590.
9. Jung R, Soondrum K, Krüger W, Neumaier M. Detection of micrometastasis through tissue-specific gene expression: its promise and problems. Recent Results Cancer Res. 2001; 158:32–39.
10. Van de Vijver MJ, Nussc R. Thc molccular biology of brcast cancer. Biochim Biophys Acta. 1991; 1072:33–50.
11. Wagener C, Breuer H. [Diagnostic significance of tumour markers in clinical chemistry. Report on the workshop conference of the German Society for Clinical Chemistry, held on November 15–17, 1979 in Schloss Auel (author's transl.)]. J Clin Chem Clin Biochem. 1980; 18:821–827.
12. Gerhard M, Juhl H, Kalthoff H, Schreiber HW, Wagener C, Neumaier M. Specific detection of carcinoembryonic antigen-expressing tumour cells in bone marrow aspirates by polymerase chain reaction. J Clin Oncol. 1994; 12:725–729.
13. Futamura M, Takagi Y, Koumura H, Kida H, Tanemura H, Shimokawa K *et al.* Spread of colorectal cancer micrometastases in regional lymph nodes by reverse transcriptase-polymerase chain reactions for carcinoembryonic antigen and cytokeratin 20. J Surg Oncol. 1998; 68:34–40.
14. Mori M, Mimori K, Inoue H, Barnard GF, Tsuji K, Nanbara S *et al.* Detection of cancer micrometastases in lymph nodes by reverse transcriptase-polymerase chain reaction. Cancer Res. 1995; 55:3417–3420.

15. Moll R, Franke WW, Schiller DL, Geiger B, Krepler R. The catalog of human cytokeratins: patterns of expression in normal epithelia, tumours and cultured cells. Cell. 1982; 31:11–24.
16. Tschentscher P, Wagener C, Neumaier M. Sensitive and specific cytokeratin 18 reverse transcription-polymerase chain reaction that excludes amplification of processed pseudogenes from contaminating genomic DNA. Clin Chem. 1997; 43:2244–2250.
17. Krüger W, Krzizanowski C, Holweg M, Stockschläder M, Kröger N, Jung R *et al.* Reverse transcriptase/polymerase chain reaction detection of cytokeratin-19 mRNA in bone marrow and blood of breast cancer patients. J Cancer Res Clin Oncol. 1996; 122:679–686.
18. Soeth E, Roder C, Juhl H, Krüger U, Kremer B, Kalthoff H. The detection of disseminated tumour cells in bone marrow from colorectal-cancer patients by a cytokeratin-20-specific nested reverse-transcriptase-polymerase-chain reaction is related to the stage of disease. Int J Cancer. 1996; 69:278–282.
19. Datta YH, Adams PT, Drobyski WR, Ethier SP, Terry VH, Roth MS. Sensitive detection of occult breast cancer by the reverse-transcriptase polymerase chain reaction. J Clin Oncol. 1994; 12:475–482.
20. Fields KK, Elfenbein GJ, Trudeau WL, Perkins JB, Janssen WE, Moscinski LC. Clinical significance of bone marrow metastases as detected using the polymerase chain reaction in patients with breast cancer undergoing high-dose chemotherapy and autologous bone marrow transplantation. J Clin Oncol. 1996; 14:1868–1876.
21. Noguchi S, Hiratsuka M, Furukawa H, Aihara T, Kasugai T, Tamura S *et al.* Detection of gastric cancer micrometastases in lymph nodes by amplification of keratin 19 mRNA with reverse transcriptase-polymerase chain reaction. Jpn J Cancer Res. 1996; 87:650–654.
22. Aihara T, Noguchi S, Ishikawa O, Furukawa H, Hiratsuka M, Ohigashi H *et al.* Detection of pancreatic and gastric cancer cells in peripheral and portal blood by amplification of keratin 19 mRNA with reverse transcriptase-polymerase chain reaction. Int J Cancer. 1997; 72:408–411.
23. Soeth E, Vogel I, Roder C, Juhl H, Marxsen J, Kruger U *et al.* Comparative analysis of bone marrow and venous blood isolates from gastrointestinal cancer patients for the detection of disseminated tumour cells using reverse transcription PCR. Cancer Res. 1997; 57:3106–3110.
24. Moll R, Lowe A, Laufer J, Franke WW. Cytokeratin 20 in human carcinomas. A new histodiagnostic marker detected by monoclonal antibodies. Am J Pathol. 1992; 140:427–447.
25. Hildebrandt M, Mapara MY, Korner IJ, Bargou RC, Moldenhauer G, Dorken B. Reverse transcriptase-polymerase chain reaction (RT-PCR)-controlled immunomagnetic purging of breast cancer cells using the magnetic cell separation (MACS) system: a sensitive method for monitoring purging efficiency. Exp Hematol. 1997; 25:57–65.
26. Gendler SJ, Spicer AP. Epithelial mucin genes. Annu Rev Physiol. 1995; 57:607–634.
27. Dearnaley DP, Ormerod MG, Sloane JP. Micrometastases in breast cancer: long-term follow-up of the first patient cohort. Eur J Cancer. 1991; 27:236–239.
28. Diel IJ, Kaufmann M, Costa SD, Holle R, von MG, Solomayer EF *et al.* Micrometastatic breast cancer cells in bone marrow at primary surgery: prognostic value in comparison with nodal status. J Natl Cancer Inst. 1996; 88:1652–1658.

29. Delsol G, Gatter KC, Stein H, Erber WN, Pulford KA, Zinne K *et al*. Human lymphoid cells express epithelial membrane antigen. Implications for diagnosis of human neoplasms. Lancet. 1984; 2:1124–1129.
30. Takahashi T, Makiguchi Y, Hinoda Y, Kakiuchi H, Nakagawa N, Imai K *et al*. Expression of MUC1 on myeloma cells and induction of HLA-unrestricted CTL against MUC1 from a multiple myeloma patient. J Immunol. 1994; 153:2102–2109.
31. Brugger W, Buhring HJ, Grunebach F, Vogel W, Kaul S, Muller R *et al*. Expression of MUC-1 epitopes on normal bone marrow: implications for the detection of micrometastatic tumour cells. J Clin Oncol. 1999; 17:1535–1544.
32. Noguchi S, Aihara T, Nakamori S, Motomura K, Inaji H, Imaoka S *et al*. The detection of breast carcinoma micrometastases in axillary lymph nodes by means of reverse transcriptase-polymerase chain reaction. Cancer. 1994; 74:1595–1600.
33. Becker RM, Darrow C, Zimonjic DB, Popescu NC, Watson MA, Fleming TP. Identification of mammaglobin B, a novel member of the uteroglobin gene family. Genomics. 1998; 54:70–78.
34. Watson MA, Dintzis S, Darrow CM, Voss LE, DiPersio J, Jensen R *et al*. Mammaglobin expression in primary, metastatic, and occult breast cancer. Cancer Res. 1999; 59:3028–3031.
35. Zach O, Kasparu H, Krieger O, Hehenwarter W, Girschikofsky M, Lutz D. Detection of circulating mammary carcinoma cells in the peripheral blood of breast cancer patients via a nested reverse transcriptase polymerase chain reaction assay for mammaglobin mRNA. J Clin Oncol. 1999; 17:2015.
36. Patton S, Gendler SJ, Spicer AP. The epithelial mucin, MUC1, of milk, mammary gland and other tissues. Biochim Biophys Acta. 1995; 1241:407–423.
37. Larocca D, Peterson JA, Urrea R, Kuniyoshi J, Bistrain AM, Ceriani RL. A Mr 46,000 human milk fat globule protein that is highly expressed in human breast tumours contains factor VIII-like domains. Cancer Res. 1991; 51:4994–4998.
38. Larocca D, Peterson JA, Walkup G, Urrea R, Ceriani RL. Cloning and sequencing of a complementary DNA encoding a Mr 70,000 human breast epithelial mucin-associated antigen. Cancer Res. 1990; 50:5925–5930.
39. Krüger WH, Jung R, Detlefsen B, Badbaran A, Renges H, Kröger N *et al*. Interference of cytokeratin-20- and mammaglobin-reverse transcriptase polymerase chain assays designed for the detection of disseminated cancer cells. Med Oncol. 2001; 18:33–38.
40. Dent GA, Civalier CJ, Brecher ME, Bentley SA. MUC1 expression in hematopoietic tissues. Am J Clin Pathol. 1999; 111:741–747.
41. Krüger W, Kröger N, Zander AR. MUC1 expression in hemopoietic tissues. J Hematother Stem Cell Res. 2000; 9:409–410.
42. Krüger W, Lohner R, Jung R, Kröger N, Zander AR. Expression of human milk fat globulin proteins in cells of haemopoietic origin. Brit J Cancer. 2000; 83:874–879.
43. Traweek ST, Liu J, Battifora H. Keratin gene expression in non-epithelial tissues. Detection with polymerase chain reaction. Am J Pathol. 1993; 142:1111–1118.
44. Jung R, Krüger W, Hosch S, Holweg M, Kroger N, Gutensohn K *et al*. Specificity of reverse transcriptase polymerase chain reaction assays designed for the detection of circulating cancer cells is influenced by cytokines in vivo and in vitro. Brit J Cancer. 1998; 78:1194–1198.
45. Jung R, Petersen K, Krüger W, Wolf M, Wagener C, Zander A *et al*. Detection of micrometastasis by cytokeratin 20 RT-PCR is limited due to stable background transcription in granulocytes. Brit J Cancer. 1999; 81:870–873.

46. Krüger W, Jung R, Kröger N, Gutensohn K, Fiedler W, Neumaier M *et al.* Sensitivity of assays designed for the detection of disseminated epithelial tumour cells is influenced by cell separation methods. Clin Chem. 2000; 46:435–436.
47. Krismann M, Todt B, Schroder J, Gareis D, Muller KM, Seeber S *et al.* Low specificity of cytokeratin 19 reverse transcriptase-polymerase chain reaction analyses for detection of hematogenous lung cancer dissemination. J Clin Oncol. 1995; 13:2769–2775.
48. Zippelius A, Kufer P, Honold G, Kollermann MW, Oberneder R, Schlimok G *et al.* Limitations of reverse-transcriptase polymerase chain reaction analyses for detection of micrometastatic epithelial cancer cells in bone marrow. J Clin Oncol. 1997; 15:2701–2708.
49. Krüger W, Datta C, Badbaran A, Tögel F, Gutensohn K, Carrero I *et al.* Immunomagnetic tumour cell selection – implications for the detection of disseminated cancer cells. Transfusion. 2000; 40:1489–1493.

Chapter 2

RNA/DNA BASED DETECTION OF MINIMAL RESIDUAL HEAD AND NECK CANCER

Ruud H. Brakenhoff

Section Tumour Biology, Department of Otolaryngology/Head-Neck Surgery Vrije Universiteit Medical Center

Abstract

The prognosis of head and neck cancer is largely determined by the radicality of treatment: residual tumour cells will grow out and develop in manifest local recurrences, regional recurrences and distant metastases. Classical diagnostic methods such as radiology and histopathology have limited sensitivities, and only by molecular techniques minimal residual cancer or disseminated tumour cells can be detected. In tissue samples containing the normal tissue counterpart of a tumour only (pre)cancer cell-specific markers can be exploited, whereas in other samples tissue-specific markers can be used. Currently, there are two main methodologies in use, one based on antigen-antibody interaction, and the other based on amplified nucleic acids. The most commonly used nucleic acid markers are mutations or alterations in tumour DNA (tumour-specific markers) or differentially expressed mRNA (tissue-specific markers). The limits of detection of these molecular assays can reach levels of a single tumour cell in a background of 2×10^7 normal cells. The assays are, however, often complex, demand a large experience and are usually laborious. Nevertheless, the data collected with these assays enable the elucidation of unexplained clinical phenomena. Further technical developments might allow implementation in clinical practice once the relevance has been assessed in large prognostic trials with long-term follow-up. In this chapter a number of the molecular assays used for (pre)cancer cell detection in head and neck cancer patients will be presented.

1. SQUAMOUS CELL CARCINOMA OF THE HEAD AND NECK

Cancer of the head and neck is the fifth most common incident cancer throughout the world. Head and neck cancer accounts for 42,000 new cases of cancer and 12,000 deaths per year in the USA. The five-year survival rates are generally about 50% to 70% (1–3). About 95% of all head and neck cancers in the western world are squamous cell carcinomas (HNSCC) (3, 4). The treatment failure of head and neck cancer is determined by local recurrences, regional recurrences in the lymph nodes above the clavicle, distant metastases and second primary tumours (5, 6). In former times the fate of the patient with head and neck cancer

K. Pantel (ed.), Micrometastasis, 19–45.

was determined by the local tumour process which rapidly destroyed the vital anatomical structures in this region (7). After the introduction of surgical techniques for resection of the tumour at the primary site, recurrence in the lymph nodes above the clavicles gained importance (8). In 1906 the neck dissection was introduced by Crile (9) as a treatment methodology for the regional lymph nodes. Improvement of surgical techniques, as well as the introduction and development of radiotherapy and chemoradiotherapy, further increased the locoregional control twofold. However, the improved locoregional control resulted in only a moderately increased survival rate of HNSCC patients, as also the rate of distant metastases increased twofold (10–14). Recently, long-term results of the treatment of HNSCC at the base of the tongue with surgery and radiotherapy were published with a median follow-up of 36 months, showing successful local control in 89% of the cases and neck control in 96% of the cases. The most common site of treatment failure was the development of distant metastases in 24% of the cases (15). These long-term results demonstrate the possibilities of modern diagnostic and therapeutic modalities. It should be mentioned, however, that the risk for locoregional recurrences strongly depends on the site and stage of the tumour, as well as the therapeutical management. For example, tumours in the larynx have a much better prognosis than tumours in the floor of the mouth mainly due to the well-defined anatomical borders of the larynx.

Lymph node metastasis is the most important mechanism in the spread of HNSCC. In general, lymph nodes are rather poor barriers to tumour cells (16), and clinical practice has shown that lymph nodes quite often appear to be a fertile soil for tumour growth. The presence of lymph node metastases is an important prognosticator in head and neck cancer. The presence of lymph node metastasis reduces the expected survival by approximately 50% (17–20). The frequency of lymph node metastasis is dependent on the site and the T stage of the tumour (see below). For example, T1, T2 and T3 oral tongue carcinomas have a risk for nodal involvement of 18%, 33% and 60% respectively, whereas T1, T2 and T3 floor of the mouth carcinomas have a risk of 38%, 65% and 71% respectively (21, 22). Not only the presence, but also the number of nodal metastases, the level in the neck, the size of the nodes and the presence of extranodal spread are important prognostic factors (19).

The neck nodes are divided into five anatomically defined levels, all of which are dissected in a comprehensive neck dissection. The lymph nodes in the different levels have different rates for metastatic involvement (21). The levels 1, 2 and 3 are more often affected by lymph node metastases than levels 4, 5 and 6 (22). Most tumours have a well-defined and predictable pattern of metastasis to the neck (23–25). For example, tumours in the anterior floor of the mouth disseminate most frequently to level 1. Many studies on this subject have been published, some deriving the data from unreliable clinical findings (26), and others from pathological reports obtained from therapeutical (27, 28), or elective neck dissections (23, 29). From the many studies published it can be derived that primary carcinomas from all sites can eventually spread to all levels of the neck (30).

Besides lymph node metastases, about 15% to 25% of the HNSCC patients develop distant metastases (19). Autopsy studies even report on a much higher incidence of distant metastases of 40% to 57% (31–33). The lungs are the most frequent site of metastases (52–60%), followed by the skeletal system (19–35%). Other localizations of metastatic deposits are the liver, mediastinum, skin, and brain (19).

Since the introduction of the TNM staging the treatment planning is based on this anatomical staging methodology. The tumours are classified from T_1 to T_4 mainly based on size of the tumour, and the lymph node metastases from N_0 to N_3 based on site, size, and number. The presence or absence of distant metastases is indicated by M_1 or M_0, respectively. The TNM stages are grouped in clinical disease Stages I–IV, with higher stages related to lower survival rates (34). Clinical T staging is based on visual inspection, computed tomography (CT)-scans and magnetic resonance imaging (MRI) of the tumour. N staging is mainly based on palpation, CT, MRI, ultrasound sonography, and ultrasound-guided fine needle aspiration cytology (USgFNAC). When surgical treatment is planned, the clinical T and N staging are confirmed by histopathological examination of the specimen resulting in a pTN classification, the current 'gold standard'. Moreover, the presence or absence of tumour in the resection margins, as well as extracapsular spread of lymph node metastases, are determined by histopathological examination. M staging is performed by radiological methods such as X-ray, scintigraphy, and ultrasound sonography.

Based on the anatomical staging, the treatment planning has largely improved. The early stages of disease (Stage I/II) are treated with ablative surgery or radiotherapy alone, while the later stages are treated with combinations of radiotherapy, surgery, and/or chemoradiotherapy. About one-third of the head and neck cancer patients presents with early stage (I and II) HNSCC, while two-thirds present with locoregional advanced disease (Stage III and IV) (35).

2. SECOND PRIMARY TUMOURS AND FIELD CANCERIZATION

Head and neck cancer patients are at relatively high risk to develop a second primary tumour (SPT) after curative treatment of the primary index tumour. SPT occur at a constant rate of 3% per year and the five-year cumulative incidence ranges from 15% to 35%. Second primary tumours are designated synchronous or metachronous dependent on whether they were diagnosed within 6 months or after 6 months after diagnosis of the index tumour, respectively. The majority of these tumours occur at different sites within the head and neck region, but also at sites like oesophagus and lungs (36–38). Second primary tumours have in general a poor prognosis, because they arise frequently at sites that are difficult to treat. The occurrence of second primary tumours is currently the major cause of treatment failure two years after treatment of early stage head and neck cancer.

In recent studies on advanced HNSCC it was shown that improved locoregional control did not result in improved survival, but in increasing rates of distant metastases and second primary tumours. In this study, 21% of the patients had developed second malignancies (15). These observations, although in selected groups of patients, underscore the increasing importance of second primary tumours in HNSCC.

It should be stressed, however, that controversy exists about the definition of second primary tumours. For the classification of second primary tumours the criteria of Warren and Gates (39), later modified by Hong *et al.* (40), are commonly used. These criteria require that both tumours are histologically malignant and that they are geographically separate and distinct. Moreover, it should be excluded that the SPT is a metastasis of the index tumour. When a second primary tumour occurs in the lung, then the differential diagnosis from a lung metastasis is often difficult. Criteria that are used to distinguish an SPT from a distant metastasis in the lung are the localization (peripheral versus central) and the time of onset after curative treatment of the first tumour. Distant metastases are usually present within two years after initial treatment (19). Lesions in the lung that occur after three years are, therefore, often designated as SPT.

When a second primary tumour occurs in the same anatomical site, the distinction with local recurrences is often difficult. As a measure of the geographical distance the minimum of two centimeters is used or, alternatively, again, the time difference of 3 years between first and second tumour. Gradually genetic information gains importance in the definition of SPT. Loss of heterozygosity (LOH) profiling or mutational analysis of both tumours can, for instance, be used to investigate their clonal relationship (see below). LOH profiling of a number of first and second primary tumours within the same individuals revealed that they often share a common clonal origin (41), and that many second primary tumours in the lung may in fact be distant metastases (42).

The aetiology of the development of SPT is not clear. The exposure of large areas of the mucosa to the same carcinogenic substances present in cigarette smoke or alcoholic beverages have led to the concept of 'field cancerization' which assumes that the entire mucous membrane of the respiratory and upper digestive tract is at risk for neoplasia (43). Recent data using molecular approaches gave new insight (see below).

Besides exposure to similar carcinogenic agents, the risk to develop second primary tumours seems to be related to an intrinsic susceptibility to cancer. Cloos *et al.* (44) have shown that HNSCC patients who have developed second malignancies have an increased mutagen sensitivity profile, indicating that they are hypersensitive for carcinogenic assaults. In a retrospective multicentre study exploring the role of mutagen sensitivity for the development of HNSCC it was found that the hypersensitive individuals who had smoked more than 25 pack-years, had a relative risk of 45 to develop HNSCC as compared to the insensitive non-smokers (45). Analysis of the mutagen sensitivity phenotype in monozygotic and dizygotic twins revealed a heritability factor of 73% (46). The elucidation of the underlying molecular mechanisms which cause this hypersensitive phenotype will be one of the challenges for the coming years. This will be particularly important for the identification of persons at a high risk to develop second malignancies since those patients can be subjected to a more intense follow-up and be enrolled in prevention trials.

To reduce the incidence of second malignancies in curatively treated HNSCC patients chemoprevention has been introduced. First results showing a beneficial effect of chemopreventive treatment on the development of second malignancies were with 13-cis-retinoic acid (40). However, most subsequent trials were less successful (47; reviewed in 48)

In conclusion, it is anticipated that improved control of the primary disease may result in an increased rate of second primary tumours. Identification of the cell biological mechanisms and the aetiology factors underlying the occurrence of second malignancies will be crucial to manage this increasing clinical problem.

3. MOLECULAR ASSESSMENT OF SURGICAL MARGINS BY MUTATED-p53

3.1 General Aspects

The success rate of surgical treatment of HNSCC patients is largely dependent on the often microscopically undetectable tumour cells that are left behind in the patient. The classical diagnostic modalities, such as histopathology and radiology, are often not sensitive enough to detect these small numbers of cells, but recent advances in molecular diagnostic methods based on tissue-specific or tumour-specific markers are currently filling this gap. Particularly in head and neck cancer a more sensitive detection of minimal residual cancer (MRC) in resection margins seems of importance, as residual tumour cells might play a crucial role in the relatively high recurrence rates observed in these patients. Local recurrences occur in about 10% to 30% of the cases even with histopathologically tumour-free surgical margins (19), and molecular analysis might improve the staging of these patients. However, the use of molecular markers is hampered by the fact that normal mucosa is present in these samples. This implies that only markers can be used that are tumour-specific, or at least not present in normal keratinocytes of the mucosa.

To date, it is widely accepted that cancer arises as a result of the accumulation of genetic alterations in oncogenes and tumour suppressor genes followed by clonal evolution. Some of these alterations occur specifically in the genes that play a crucial role in the normal behaviour of the cell, but often these changes appear in less crucial sequences and are therefore a mere reflection of the genetic instability of the tumours (49). Hence, tumour cells harbour specific clonal genetic changes that can be used as molecular markers for the detection of (pre)cancer cells in clinical samples. The choice of a particular marker or assay depends on the necessary sensitivity and specificity of the assay, the origin of the clinical sample and the laboriousness of the assay. The introduction of *in vitro* nucleic acid amplification methods, most notably the polymerase chain reaction (PCR) that enables amplification of minute amounts of DNA more than a million-fold, triggered the development of novel sensitive technologies for the detection of tumour cells by molecular markers. When directed towards genetic abnormalities/characteristics specific for tumours, PCR-based methods might be powerful tools to detect low numbers of tumour cells in the presence of an excess of normal cells (50, 51). Consequently, an improvement of the sensitivity of detecting residual or disseminated disease can be obtained. In the first part, below, molecular assays using DNA markers are discussed, specifically exploited to detect cells clonally related to the tumour in surgical margins of HNSCC patients to elucidate the basis of the unexplained local recurrences in histological-tumour-free margins, as well as the origination of second primary tumours. In the second part, highly sensitive RT-PCR assays will be discussed making use of tissue-specific expressed RNA markers for the detection of disseminated cancer cells in lymph nodes, blood, and bone marrow.

The first genetic progression model was described for colorectal cancer in which the accumulation of genetic alterations had been demonstrated (49). The transitional stages of this model, ranging from normal epithelium, via adenoma to invasive carcinoma and metastases, are associated with mutations affecting oncogenes (e.g., K-ras) and tumour suppressor genes (e.g., p53). Moreover, it was shown that at these various stages the cells often display genetic instability which can be observed at the DNA level as amplifications, deletions, or alterations of DNA repeat sequences, known as microsatellites (52). A variant of this sequential genetic progression model was later described for squamous cell carcinoma of the head and neck (53). In this model it was shown that the histological changes recognized as hyperplasia and dysplasia (mild, moderate, and severe) run in parallel to genetic changes. Early changes in progression were loss of heterozygosity of 9p (p14/p16 genes), 3p (gene unknown), and 17p (p53).

A genetic event that appears to be of significance in the progression of many tumour types, including HNSCC, is loss of the p53 tumour suppressor gene, either through allelic deletion and/or mutation (54–56). Alterations in the p53 gene are an integral part of cancer progression in almost all types of human cancer and the assumption that they precede the stage of invasive cancer favours their use as marker for cancer staging.

Mutated p53 has successfully been used as marker to detect cells clonally related to the tumour in various tissues and body fluids (57–59). In recent years, numerous methods have been described for the detection of DNA with point mutations in a background of normal DNA (tumour cells within normal cells in clinical samples) among which the plaque hybridization assay (57), mutant-allele specific amplification (MASA [60]), oligonucleotide ligation assay (OLA [61]), POINT-EXACCT (a modified oligonucleotide ligation assay [62]), enriched restriction fragment length polymorphism PCR (RFLP-PCR [63–66]) and very recently also digital PCR (67). In a previous study in 25 head and neck cancer patients, molecular assessment of surgical margins using p53 mutations as marker for detecting cells clonally related to the tumour appeared to be superior to histopathological staging (68). This pilot study demonstrated the potential of these molecular approaches. Moreover, in this pilot study the data were shown to be clinically relevant as it correctly predicted local recurrences in patients with molecular-positive surgical margins. Therefore, we initiated a clinical trial with approximately 200 head and neck cancer patients for the assessment of cells clonally related to the tumour using p53 mutations as marker for analysis of resection margins, and E48 gene expression for assessment of lymph nodes, blood and bone marrow (see below). In addition, we evaluated the suitability of p53 mutations as molecular marker, and explored a number of various DNA assays to detect p53-mutated DNA in a background of normal DNA. As yet, the plaque hybridization assay is still the most reliable, quantitative and robust method for tumour cell detection using p53 mutations as marker. The plaque hybridization assay will be discussed in detail.

3.2 Identification of Mutations in the p53 Gene

Sequencing of the p53 gene should in theory be straightforward, but is in practice rather complex. This statement underlies the large reported differences in the mutational frequencies of p53: a considerable number of these differences can be explained by the method used for sequencing. Most researchers currently use direct DNA cycle sequencing, either with fluorescent chromophores or radioactive labels. In addition, also the p53 GeneChip assay (Affymetrix, Santa Clara, CA 95051, USA [68]) and MALDI-TOF mass spectrometry (69) are being used for (p53) sequencing. For allele discrimination in blood samples these methods seem equivalent, but for sequencing DNA derived from tumour tissue the method used becomes more critical. The number of tumour cells is often low in a tumour biopsy and the DNA of relative poor quality that might result in the missing of mutations or the introduction of artificial mutations. Particularly, sequencing of DNA isolated from archival paraffin-embedded tumour tissue is difficult and leads easily to artificial results (70; and own unpublished data). In general, both fluorescent and radioactive cycle sequencing are based on Sangers dideoxynucleotide method. As tumour samples are always contaminated by stroma, neoplastic areas in sections of the tumour need to be micro-dissected before DNA is isolated. Subsequently, the appropriate fragment, usually the domain encoded by exons 5–9, of the p53 gene is amplified. A large fragment of 1.8 kb containing the exons 5–9 or the separate exons can be amplified on DNA isolated from frozen specimen. For sequencing of DNA isolated from archival paraffin material smaller fragments need to be amplified. None of the present methods for mutation sequencing in tumour DNA is 100% reliable, and it is therefore important to be critical about sequencing data published. In fact, to prevent ambiguous results each mutation should formally be checked by independent (non-sequencing) methods such as differential hybridization or oligonucleotide ligation assay. When extremely high or low mutational frequencies (see below) are reported, the data should be interpreted with caution, in particular when independent proof was not included.

3.3 Suitability of p53 Mutations as a Molecular Marker

There are a number of criteria determining whether a molecular marker is reliable (71). First, the molecular marker should be specific for tumour cells or cells with cancer-related genetic alterations such that it correctly distinguishes between normal cells and (pre)cancer cells. Second, to qualify as a clonal marker, a genetic alteration should precede or occur at the stage of invasive cancer and be preserved during tumour progression and metastasis. And third, the marker has to be broadly applicable – i.e. the marker must be present in a large part of the study population. It has been firmly established by numerous studies that mutations in the p53 gene meet the first criterion, including HNSCC. The position in the genetic progression model of HNSCC supports its suitability as molecular tumour marker (53, 55, 72).

The suitability of p53 mutations as a clonal marker (usually determined by mutation screening of lymph node metastases) is being debated, and literature on this issue yields conflicting data. In a number of studies the clonal stability of p53 mutations in HNSCC tumour progression was confirmed (73, 74), whereas in other studies it could not be demonstrated (75–77) reported figures ranging from 100% concordancy (73) to a mere 25% concordancy (77). We compared known p53 mutations of 23 HNSCC tumours, detected by direct radioactive cycle sequencing and confirmed by plaque assay, with the p53 mutations of 25 matched lymph node metastases and 10 distant metastases (of 7 tumours). In all cases, concordant mutations were found between tumour and (lymph node) metastases or absence of mutations (78). These findings support the idea that p53 is closely associated with tumour progression: p53 mutations develop before lymph node metastasis and are maintained during clonal outgrowth.

Currently the major limitation of mutated p53-based detection of rare tumour cells in HNSCC patients is that p53 mutations are present in only 50% to 60% of the head and neck cancers. Its applicability is, therefore, limited. Recently, Kropveld *et al.* described a mutational frequency of almost 100% in HNSCC using p53 transcript sequencing (79). To increase the frequency of mutations in our patient group, we analysed the exons 2, 3, 4, 10, and 11 of the p53 gene of 21 HNSCC tumours that had no mutation in exons 5–9 by radioactive cycle sequencing. We found two additional mutations, one in exon 4 and one in exon 3, leading to an additional mutational frequency of 5% in the study population. These mutations were confirmed by plaque assay. We estimate that we miss 10% of the mutations based on unexplained overexpression of (mutated?) p53 in tumour biopsies, and sequencing of RNA. The final percentage would then be approximately 60% to 80%. Knowing that 10% to 20% of HNSCC is related to human papillomavirus infection that causes alternative p53 inactivation, it seems that in all head and neck cancers the p53 pathway is inactivated, and in the majority of cases via mutation.

A drawback of p53 mutations as marker is the variety of mutations over the gene that necessitates sequencing of all individual tumours, but which also makes it very difficult to find simple and sensitive assays for tumour cell detection (see below). On the other hand, the variety reduces technical artefacts such as carry-over contamination.

Summarized, p53 mutations appear to be suitable tumour-specific markers, or at least suitable markers to detect cells clonally related to the tumour, that appear to occur before the formation of metastases in HNSCC. Drawbacks are the frequency, which is approximately 60% to 80% in HNSCC, and the variety of mutations that makes it more difficult to set up simple assays for tumour cell detection.

3.4 Tumour Cell Detection by the Plaque Hybridization Assay

During the last decades, numerous elegant methods of tumour cell detection have been developed. It is not possible to review all the various assays extensively. Important considerations of a suitable assay are (1) sensitivity and specificity, (2) robustness particularly in relation to the variety of mutations in the p53 gene and (3) reliability and (4) laboriousness. Depending on the (experimental) question also, quantitative aspects might play a role. As an example, it cannot be excluded that in minimal residual cancer monitoring the risk for recurrence or metastasis is related to the number of tumour cells in the clinical sample. Only after well-performed clinical studies with long-term follow-up and using quantitative assays can this question be addressed, and therefore for the time being quantitative assays are used.

To detect tumour cells using K-ras mutations as marker numerous optimized, quantitative assays are available as the mutations involve only a few codons. However, for p53 mutations as marker the mutational spectrum is very variable, which makes it difficult to find assays which are sensitive, specific, robust, and quantitative. For these reasons, we have chosen the plaque hybridization assay as the gold standard. Our method has been slightly modified from the technique reported by Sidransky *et al.* (57). In short, on basis of the p53 gene sequence of the tumour DNA, a mutant-specific and corresponding wild-type-specific oligonucleotide are selected. In general, 17-mer oligonucleotides are selected centrally across the mutation on the target strand, an important condition being that they do not contain a dC nucleotide at the 5′-end as these are very difficult to label by polynucleotide kinase (80). In theory, there might be thermodynamically more favourable locations for the mutated base, resulting in a larger difference in melting temperature between the two oligonucleotides, but in practice the position around the centre usually fulfils the requirements of discrimination. Using DNA from the specimen of interest as template, the p53 gene (exons 5–9 or specific exons) is amplified by PCR and cloned into lambda phages. These are infected on host bacteria and the clones (plaques) transferred to nitrocellulose membranes. The plaques are analysed by differential hybridization with the radioactively labelled tumour-specific and wild-type-specific oligonucleotides as probes. Obviously, proper positive (primary tumour DNA) and negative (wild-type DNA) controls are included. The hybridization solution initially described was rather complex (57), but a regular 6 × SSC, 0.1% salmon sperm DNA (only included during prehybridization) and 5 × Denhardts also works well (40). Hybridization takes place during 18 hours at 11 degrees Celsius below the melting temperature of (one of) the probes, followed by three initial wash steps with 6 × SSC at the hybridization temperature and one final stringent wash step at 1–5 degrees Celsius below the melting temperature.

As each plaque contains identical phages with only wild-type or mutant DNA strands, the number of plaques hybridizing with the mutant oligonucleotide divided by the number of plaques hybridizing with the wild-type oligonucleotide is a reliable measure of the tumour cell DNA load in the original sample. At this point, we have added the confirmation of mutant positive plaques to identify false-positive signal. When the number of plaques hybridizing with the mutant probe is low (between 1 to 5), the signal is confirmed by classical rescreening; the positive plaque is stabbed from the agar, replated and rescreened (as example of the results see Figure 1).

In summary, the plaque assay is quantitative, well-controllable, highly reproducible and very robust. Notwithstanding the variety of p53 mutations, the assay never failed in our hands, although some particular mutations are more difficult to discriminate from wild type as others. The major drawback is the laboriousness of the assay, and it is suitable only in the experimental setting. Implementation of this assay in regular clinical care will not be possible.

3.5 Alternative Methods Using Point Mutations as Marker

As mentioned before, the plaque assay is among numerous methods that are based on point-mutation detection in (clinical) samples, some of which have only very recently been developed and would be more rapid and less laborious. Alternative methods are MASA, OLA, POINT-EXACCT, rolling-circle amplification, denaturing-HPLC, RFLP-PCR, REMS-PCR (restriction endonuclease-mediated selection), PCR-SSCP (single stranded conformation polymorphism) and digital PCR. A more detailed description of these techniques is described in (81) and references therein. A number of these methods have been explored for the analysis of heterozygotes based on point mutations, but lack sensitivity and specificity for use in minimal cancer detection. Particularly, techniques based on the different behaviour of mismatch duplex DNA molecules in various (electrophoretic) separation systems such as denaturing-HPLC, PCR-SSCP and others are usually too insensitive to detect mutant DNA strands in a large excess of wild-type DNA strands. Most other techniques fail also on the basis of the variety of p53 mutations. Sensitivity and specificity strongly depend on the location and type of mutation and, therefore, differ between assays.

Still, the ultimate assay that can exploit a large variety of point mutations as marker, which is as robust but less laborious than the plaque assay, has not yet been described. However, when large prognostic studies might indicate the benefit of molecular staging by screening surgical margins for (pe)cancer cells, improved techniques need to be developed as the plaque assay cannot be implemented in clinical care.

3.6 Problems and Pitfalls Using Point Mutations as Marker

3.6.1 Unwanted-positive Results

Assays using point mutations as marker need stringent control measures to prevent unwanted- or false-positive signal. Unwanted-positive means in this context that the mutated DNA was present in the sample, but its presence is not in line with the clinical correlations. False-positive means that mutated DNA was not present in the sample, and the signal was derived as a result from technical artefacts. In studies on residual head and neck cancer in surgical margins, tumour cell (DNA) contamination can occur: (1) in the operating room and (2) during histopathological processing of the samples. Besides contamination with tumour cells, also contamination with DNA might occur. Particularly, since it was noticed that tumour DNA can be found in the serum (82, 83), it needs to be considered that tumour DNA floats at least through the lymph. Moreover, necrotic tumours might cause tumour DNA contamination via the saliva. Several precautions should be taken in every step to prevent at least artificial contamination by tumour cells or tumour cell DNA. For example, before sampling resection margins in the operation room, the operating field needs to be extensively rinsed and the instruments changed. Similarly, the working area of the pathologist is cleaned before the lymph nodes are dissected from the surgical specimen, and the dissection instruments of the pathologist are decontaminated between lymph node preparations in 0.1 M HCl and PBS (phosphate buffered saline).

3.6.2 False-positive Results

A well-known drawback of very sensitive PCR assays is carry-over contamination. By contamination of a clinical sample with amplimers of another sample after PCR amplification, false-positive results might occur. A detailed evaluation of these problems, and solutions to prevent them, have been described previously (81).

A second source of false-positive results in the plaque assay or any other assays using point mutations as marker could also be caused by the enzyme that is used to amplify the DNA: a thermostable DNA polymerase. It is known that the used enzyme (in our case, Taq polymerase) produces spontaneous single-base substitution errors at reported frequencies of 1/9,000 nucleotides polymerized (84, 85). However, the probability to detect a misincorporated base as a false-positive result depends mainly on the number of template molecules introduced in the PCR reaction, and much less on the Taq error. When more than 500,000 template molecules are introduced (corresponding to approximately 250 nanograms of chromosomal DNA), Taq errors can be neglected. However, when (archival) stained and fixed DNA is analysed for point mutations, the error frequencies considerably increase (70): however, in these cases, not by Taq misincorporation, but merely by chemical damage of the bases (Nieuwenhuis *et al.*, submitted).

3.7 Initial Clinical Results

In total, 179 patients have been enrolled in our study on molecular analysis of surgical margins of whom 143 were histologically radical. From 128 of these 143 patients, all material was available. In 69 patients we could detect a p53 mutation. Using the identified mutation in the p53 gene, mutated DNA (cells clonally related to the tumour) was detected using the plaque hybridization assay. A typical example is shown in Figure 1. The data were coupled to the clinical outcome. In total we found 47 of 69 patients with mutated-p53 in the surgical margins. Subsequently, we analysed the margins of all positive cases by immunostaining and molecular analysis to find the pathobiological source of the mutated-p53. Only in two cases we found tumour. However, in 10 of 47 cases we found tumour-related precancerous mucosal lesions in the resection margins that explained the p53-mutated DNA (the p53 mutations were identical to mutations found in the tumours). Histologically all lesions were graded as dysplasia ranging from mild to severe. Although this might have been expected as mutated p53 overexpression had been described earlier in tumour-adjacent mucosa (86, 87), it had not been described in resection margins that are often one or even more centimetres at distance. Particularly, the observation that the mutations were identical to the mutation in the tumour proved a clonal relationship, and the tumour relatedness had not been established firmly either. The presence of these large lesions in the resection margins indicated a contiguous mutated-p53 field of mucosal epithelium (see Figure 2). These lesions (genetically altered mucosal lesions or 'fields') might represent the phenomenon of 'field cancerization' (43).

As only part of the head and neck cancers show a p53 mutation, and p53 mutations (or at least accompanying 17p LOH) are not the earliest changes, we could not exclude that we only detected part of the tumour-related genetically altered fields surrounding HNSCC. Therefore, it was decided to perform a comprehensive analysis using the earliest genetic alterations (9p, 3p, 17p).

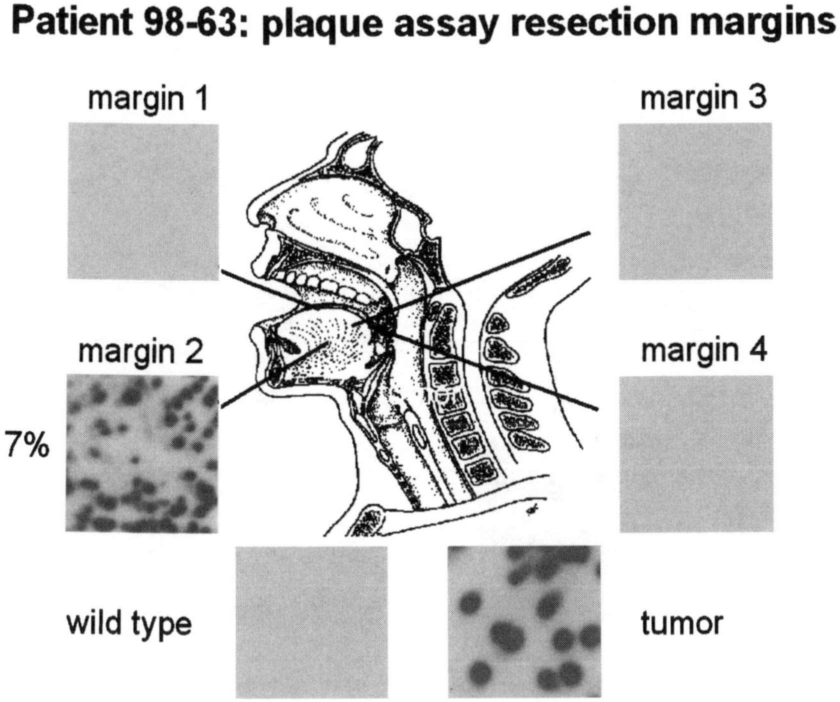

Figure 1. Patient 98-63, a male of 75 years, presented with a T1N0 tumour at the tongue and was treated by surgery. The resection margins were histologically tumour-free. The tumour DNA was sequenced for p53 mutations. In exon 8 codon 267 a CGG>GGG (Arg>Gly) mutation was found. The margins were screened by the tumour-specific mutation using tumour DNA and wild-type DNA as positive and negative controls, respectively. Margin 2 contained 7% tumour-DNA. The patient developed a local recurrence after 11 months.

4. DETECTION OF 'FIELDS' USING MICROSATELLITES AS MARKER

4.1 Genetic Alterations Detected by Microsatellites

Besides the specific changes in tumour suppressor genes and oncogenes, cancer cells are genetically unstable and display extensive chromosomal changes, including amplifications, duplications, deletions, and translocations. Some of these changes can be determined by allele-specific markers such as microsatellites, as these markers allow distinction of maternal and paternal alleles. Microsatellites are small repetitive sequences that are often highly polymorphic in the population. By PCR amplification and subsequent electrophoretic separation, the maternal and paternal alleles can be distinguished, at least when the

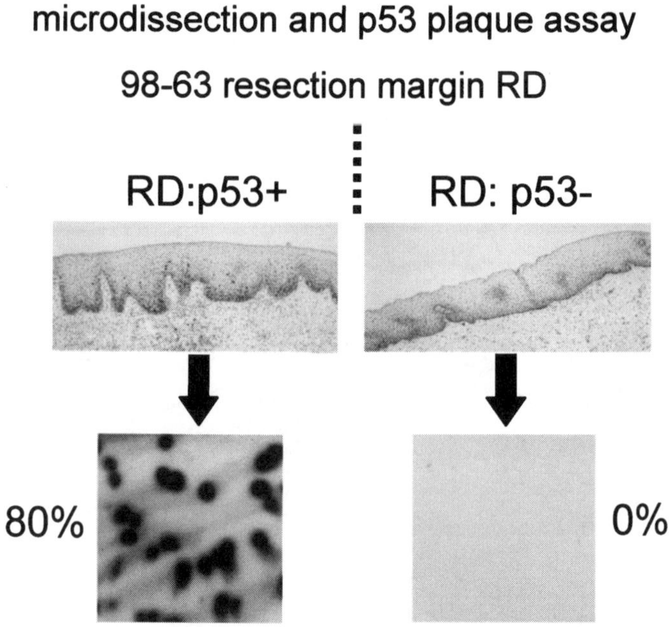

Figure 2. The paraffin-embedded tumour and margins from the resection specimen of patient 98-63 were stained by anti–p53 DO7. The tumour showed mutated-p53 overexpression. In one margin (margin RA) an intensely stained mucosal precursor lesion was seen that had not been resected completely. Molecular analysis showed that the mutation in the precursor lesion was identical to the mutation in the tumour. All paraffin sections were histopathologically reviewed without previous knowledge on the molecular data. Margin RA was graded as mild dysplasia. More detailed genetic profiling of DNA from tumour, local recurrence, and resection margins indicated that the local recurrence arose from the unresected mucosal precursor lesion (Tabor et al., *submitted).*

number of repeats differs between the two alleles (the marker is then called 'informative'). Originally these markers were exploited for genetic analysis of tumour DNA. The loss of a specific marker in tumour DNA is usually considered as the hallmark of the loss of a specific tumour suppressor gene. Loss of the locus is thought to be the second step in the complete inactivation of both copies of a tumour suppressor gene, one allele inactivated by mutation and one allele inactivated by loss (88). In practice, tumour DNA is compared to normal DNA (usually isolated from blood lymphocytes) for many different microsatellite markers. The loss of a particular allele in a clinical sample is called loss of heterozygosity (LOH) and results from allelic deletion, duplication, or amplification.

The genetic instability of tumours can also be reflected in changes in the length of the microsatellite (shifts), indicative of microsatellite instability (MSI).

MSI is characterized as a tumour-specific change of length in a microsatellite due to either insertion or deletion of repeating units, when compared to matching normal DNA (89). MSI has been described in numerous human neoplasms, but is particularly common in most hereditary non-polyposis colorectal carcinoma (HNPCC) and in a proportion of sporadic colorectal tumours (90, 91).

Usually LOH is calculated as the ratio between short allele-normal/long allele-normal and short allele-tumour/long allele-tumour, or in formula (Sn:Ln)/(St:Lt). Normally, an LOH is scored when 50% of the allele is lost in the tumour (score <0.5 or >2), but other researchers use less strict criteria. Borderline data are solved by more precise microdissection. Using this quantitation, also corrections for stutter can be made. Stutter occurs as a result of Taq polymerase slippage and causes representation of a number of fragments that differ in repeat units: a 120 bp CA repeat will show a 120, 118, 116, and 114 bp fragment, while the second allele may show a 118, 116, 114, and 112 fragment. From a particular marker, the relative contribution to the stutter bands is calculated from a non-informative sample, and used to calculate the relative abundance of the second allele to the first stutter band of the first allele. By this method, much more information can be deduced with larger panels of markers. Although LOH analysis is not a sensitive method for tumour cell (DNA) detection, it is a very suitable technique combined with micro-dissection to screen for genetic alterations in the mucosa of resection margins of head and neck cancer patients.

Based on previous data and data in the literature, Tabor *et al.* (92) from our group performed a comprehensive analysis for genetically altered lesions surrounding HNSCC using LOH at 15 microsatellite markers on chromosome arms 9p, 3p, 17p, 8p, 13q, 18q as well as p53 mutations as genetic markers to determine (1) the presence, (2) tumour relatedness, (3) extension, and (4) persistence of these lesions. Our data showed that in 10/28 patients tumour-related genetically altered lesions could be detected when four biopsies were taken and screened, one in every quadrant around the tumour. In 7/10 (overall 7/28: 25%) the genetically altered field extended into the resection margins. Using p53 mutations as marker, it was demonstrated that the lesions persisted over time for at least 1.5 years (92). All margins and mucosal biopsies were reviewed by histopathological examination, and in all genetically altered lesions dysplasia was seen ranging from mild to severe. In contrast, in only 50% of the lesions graded as mild dysplasia genetic alterations could be found. In one case, a local recurrence was observed which appeared to have developed within the tumour-related field, graded as mild dysplasia. These data strongly support the theory that HNSCC arise in precursor lesions that can extend over several centimetres. A subclone in the lesion develops into a tumour, which is diagnosed and surgically removed. In 25% of the cases, the precursor lesion stays behind and is left untreated which leads, in some cases, to local recurrences and SPTs that should in fact both be addressed as 'Second Field Tumours' (93). Both frequency and time frame of progression to invasive carcinoma are unknown as yet. This concept of contiguous genetically altered fields also explains at least in part the concept of 'field cancerization', originally proposed by Slaughter *et al.* (43).

5. MOLECULAR MARKERS FOR DETECTION OF DISSEMINATED TUMOUR CELLS

5.1 Immunocytochemical Assays

Since 1869, circulating tumour cells have been noticed by clinicians and investigators (94). However, the number of circulating tumour cells is in general low, and only since the development of techniques with a high sensitivity, has this research area obtained increasingly more attention. A major breakthrough was the immunocytology that was exploited in large numbers of studies with high clinical impact (95–97). In a recent study, Braun *et al.* (97) demonstrated the clinical significance of bone marrow assessment for patients with breast cancer. In breast cancer the presence of axillary lymph node metastases is an important prognostic indicator. However, even in the node-negative patients up to 30% develop distant metastases, whereas 40% of the node-positive patients survive ten years or more. The presence of tumour cells in the bone marrow was very significantly correlated to a poor survival and disease-free survival. Particularly for the patients with no lymph node metastases, it was suggested to use the bone marrow status as criterion to select patients for chemotherapy (97).

Similar immunocytochemical techniques have been exploited for detection of disseminated tumour cells in head and neck cancer patients as well. However, there are only two reports that describe clinical significance (98, 99), suggesting that there are disseminated tumour cells in the bone marrow that are related to clinical outcome. Gath and Brakenhoff (99) performed an immunocytochemical assay using the monoclonal antibody (mAb) A45/B-B3 which recognizes, among others, cytokeratins 8, 18, and 19. These antigens are highly expressed in large numbers of HNSCC as shown by positive staining on cryosections of the primary tumour (100). One million cells isolated from the bone marrow were screened for cytokeratin-positive cells by immunocytochemistry (for more details see below). Until now, 149 patients were screened with the described assay. Disseminated cells were detected in 30 patients (20.1%) with a frequency of 1–207 cells per million. In one case, manifest metastasis in the bone marrow of a patient was predicted by the presence of disseminated cells identified by the described immunocytological assay. The metastasis was not detectable by conventional radiological methods, but was later confirmed by histopathological examination at autopsy when the patient had died. This observation, although in only one case, indicates that at least a subset of these cells has the potency to develop into manifest distant metastases. From 57 patients the clinical follow-up was determined ranging from 3 to 36 months (medium 17 months). In approximately 70% of the patients with immunocytochemically positive cells in the bone marrow a tumour relapse occurred, whereas in comparison only around 35% of the patients with a negative bone marrow status relapsed. A Kaplan-Meier analysis showed a statistically significant difference between patients with or without immunocytochemically positive cells in the bone marrow in relation to disease-free survival.

Another study using immunostaining techniques showed similar results (98). In this study a mAb directed against cytokeratin 19 was used for the identification of epithelial cells in bone marrow. Epithelial cells were detected in bone marrow aspirates in 41 of 108 HNSCC patients (37%). In clinical Stage I disease tumour cells were detected in 26.3% of the patients, whereas in Stage IV disease almost twice as many patients presented with tumour cells in the bone marrow. Follow-up data with a mean follow-up time of 25 months (range 4–52 months) were available for 73 patients. The presence of epithelial cells at the time of primary treatment appeared to indicate a significant higher risk for development of local or distant recurrences ($p=0.01$). Furthermore, the study revealed that patients presenting with bone marrow tumour cells showed a significant shorter disease-free interval than those without ($p=0.002$).

Although both studies support the idea that bone marrow analysis might have impact for the staging of HNSCC patients, large prospective trials with long-term follow-up focused on survival, disease-free survival, locoregional recurrence-free survival and distant metastasis-free survival, including multivariate analysis, have not been reported to date.

5.2 E48 RT-PCR Assay

Particularly, the laboriousness of the immunocytochemical assays and the development of the (RT)-PCR technique triggered the exploration of novel methodologies for rare tumour cell detection. Most RT-PCR methods for the detection of tumour cells from solid tumours make use of differentially expressed transcripts present in the normal tissue and retained in the malignant cells, but absent in the clinical sample of interest. It should be realized that the frequencies of tumour cells in bone marrow and blood are very low as deduced from the immunocytochemistry studies, ranging from 1 in 10^5 (breast cancer) to 1 in 10^7 (head and neck cancer). This means that the techniques exploited have to reach very high levels of sensitivity. Using the E48 antigen (human Ly-6D) as marker, we were able to detect reproducibly a single cell in a 7 ml tube of blood, corresponding to $2–7 \times 10^7$ white blood cells, but it demanded a large investment in time to get all variables controlled. The E48 antigen is abundantly expressed on the target tissue (squamous cells) and not illegitimately expressed on blood or bone marrow cells (101). RNA was isolated by hypo-osmotic lysis of red blood cells and RNAzol. Reverse transcription of 5 micrograms total RNA was performed using a gene-specific antisense primer and quadruplicate PCR amplification. Subsequently, the amplimers were run on an agarose electrophoretic gel, Southern blotted and hybridised to the E48 cDNA as probe (Figure 3).

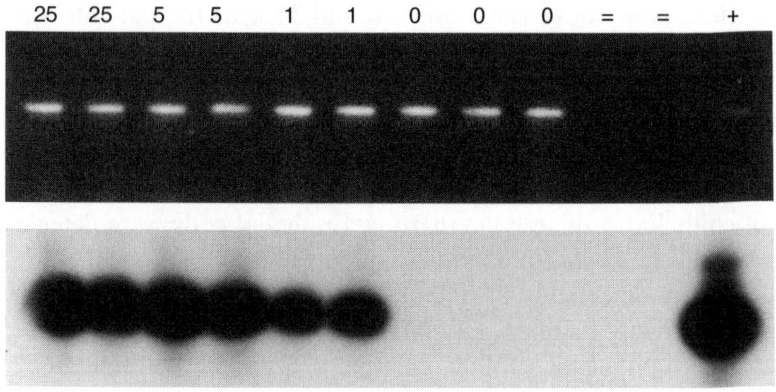

Figure 3. UM-SCC-22A cells (25, 5 ,1, and 0) were seeded in 7 ml of blood taken from a healthy volunteer. RNA was isolated and an E48 RT-PCR assay performed on 5 μg of total RNA. The Abelson housekeeping gene was used as control for the quality of the RNA (band visualized after electrophoretic gel separation at the upper panel). After blotting and hybridization, the E48 signal is seen in the lower panel. Even a single cell could be detected in 7 ml of blood (2–7 × 10^7 white blood cells) in duplicate experiments.

The detection level of a single cell per 7 ml of blood cannot be reached with DNA markers. The amount of RNA isolated from 7 ml of blood is approximately 26 micrograms. The white blood cell count in blood is on average 2–7 × 10^7 per 7 ml which corresponds to 1 picogram total RNA/cell. One HNSCC cell, however, contains 10–20 picograms of RNA per cell. Our detection limit was 1 HNSCC cell/2–7 × 10^7 white blood cells, which corresponds to 15 picograms HNSCC RNA/26 micrograms white blood cell RNA. These calculations show that at least a factor of 10 × in sensitivity is gained by the differences in RNA content between nucleated blood cells (particularly lymphocytes) and squamous cancer cells. When using DNA markers, this particular advantage will be lost, and a lot of DNA has to be tested to reach these high levels of sensitivity as 26 micrograms of genomic DNA corresponds to 0.24 × 10^7 blood cells. When sensitivities of 1 cell per 10^7 white blood cells need to be reached by DNA markers, enrichment techniques like positive and negative immunoselection become much more important.

Using the described E48 RT-PCR assay, we screened both blood and bone marrow samples of non-cancer controls and HNSCC patients. In non-cancer controls both blood and bone marrow were negative for all samples tested. It should be noted that when we tried to increase the sensitivity further using more active enzymes (AmpliTaq Gold: Applied Biosystems), a few samples became slightly positive. With our routine procedure using AMV reverse transcriptase and AmpliTaq, all 40 non-cancer controls tested remained negative. It is beyond the scope of this chapter to discuss the numerous technical problems related to this type of highly sensitive RT-PCR assay. Many of the technical problems related to sensitivity, specificity, variation between methodologies and reagents, and carry-over contamination have been discussed in (81).

In an initial pilot trial we showed that 35% of the HNSCC patients showed signal in the bone marrow and only 10% in the blood (101). To establish the clinical significance of the molecular bone marrow status we performed a larger trial. Again, one aspirate was taken from the iliac crest and analysed by E48 RT-PCR. In total 76 patients were enrolled who presented with a primary tumour, mainly Stages III and IV, and were treated by surgery often in combination with post-operative radiotherapy. Of these 76 patients, 27 were positive (36%). However, the positive bone marrow status was not associated with poor outcome in Kaplan-Meier analysis, neither for survival nor disease-free survival. When we focused on patients with more than three lymph node metastases (who have a risk of 50% to develop distant metastases), however, we were able to distinguish a high-risk and low-risk group based on the E48 RT-PCR bone marrow status. This strongly suggests that there are disseminated tumour cells in the bone marrow that might play a role in staging in clinical decision-making. However, this seems only to be relevant for patients who have more than three lymph node metastases: a large tumour load in the body. Currently these data seem less strong than the immunocytochemical data as presented so far. The discrepancies might be explained by the single aspiration we analysed versus the double aspirations used in the study presented by Gath and Brakenhoff, and the use of a different technique and marker (99). The E48 antigen is highly and homogeneously expressed on >90% of the tumours as assessed by Real-Time O-RT-PCR analysis (see below), but the expression on disseminated single tumour cells might be much lower. A trial combining double-sided aspiration as well as E48 RT-PCR and immunocytochemistry is currently being performed to solve the question whether disseminated tumour cells in bone marrow are of prognostic relevance. We will answer the question concerning single-sided or double-sided aspiration, and whether immunocytochemistry or E48 RT-PCR show the most clinically significant data.

5.3 Quantitative (Real-Time) E48 RT-PCR for Molecular Staging of the Neck

The apparent suitability of E48 RT-PCR for detection of disseminated cancer cells in bone marrow suggested that the same method might be suitable for the analysis of minimal cancer in lymph nodes and lymph node aspirates. Patients with T1/2 in the oral cavity or oropharynx and a clinically negative neck (no palpable enlarged lymph nodes that might harbour metastases) can be treated by transoral excision of the tumour. However, a clinically negative neck has a risk of 30% to 40% to harbour occult lymph node metastases. Using ultrasound-guided fine needle aspiration cytology (USgFNAC), the neck nodes can be aspirated and the aspirates cytologically screened for tumour cells. The false-negative rate of USgFNAC is approximately 20% which justifies a wait-and-see policy for the neck when there is a strict follow-up of the neck, preferably by USgFNAC, and the salvage rates by delayed neck treatment is high. Recently, we reported the long-term clinical results of this policy showing that a wait-and-see policy for the neck is justified (102).

To further improve the clinical results it is desirable to reduce the false-negative rate of USgFNAC. There are theoretically three causes that might explain false-negative USgFNAC: (1) tumour-containing lymph nodes do not fulfil the radiological criteria for aspiration (diameter of >3 to 4 mm) or tumour-containing enlarged lymph nodes are not aspirated, (2) only the tumour-free part of a tumour-containing lymph node is aspirated (sampling error), or (3) inconclusive cytology. With respect to cause 3, in 20% of the USgFNAC the quality of the preparations does not allow accurate cytological evaluation. Using E48 RT-PCR on aspirate residues, we might improve cytological screening in these cases, and might even improve the sensitivity of cytological screening. However, when we exploited the E48 RT-PCR on lymph nodes, we noticed an unwanted low level of positive signal on samples from non-cancer controls (it was not false-positive). Moreover, we wanted to have additional information with respect to the number of cells in the aspirate, the presence and number of HNSCC cells in the aspirate, and be able to correct for heterogeneity of E48 expression in the tumour. Therefore, the assay was developed further into a quantitative Real-Time RT-PCR assay that could be exploited to detect minimal disease in lymph nodes and lymph node aspirate residues. Quantitative assessment of transcripts of the house keeping gene porphobilinogen deaminase (PBGD) was used to quantify the number of cells in the aspirate residue. Quantitative assessment of E48 transcripts was set up to detect and quantify the number of HNSCC cells in the aspirate residue. The assay using both markers was linear over a 5 log range, with a correlation coefficient >0.99. A serial dilution of RNA from cell line UM-SCC-22A is used as calibration curve. The limit of detection was one to five UM-SCC-22A cells in 2×10^6 peripheral blood mononuclear cells. First, 47 micro-dissected HNSCC were screened to test heterogeneity of E48 expression. In 6 tumours the E48/PBGD ratios were below 5% UM-SCC-22A equivalents that were considered as the lowest level of expression to allow appropriate sensitive measurement. The majority of tumours showed E48/PBGD ratios >50% relative to UM-SCC-22A. Sensitivity and specificity of the E48/PBGD Q-RT-PCR assay was tested on 10 aspirate residues of non-cancer controls and 16 cytologically positive aspirate residues of HNSCC patients and were both 100%, although the number of cases tested was limited. Finally, 205 lymph node aspirate residues of 58 patients (with E48/PBGD ratios in the tumour between 5% and 400% relative to UM-SCC-22A) were tested by the E48/PBGD Q-RT-PCR assay. The number of aspirates that were not evaluable by cytological examination could be reduced by 60%. Moreover, we upstaged 6 patients from N0 to N1 based on the molecular analysis which was in 3 cases histologically/clinically confirmed (102). The data indicate the potential of these techniques to complement routine methods like cytology and histology. Currently the same quantitative RT-PCR test is exploited to screen for residual cancer cells in lymph nodes.

6. CONCLUSION AND FUTURE DIRECTIONS

In the past few years, much progress has been made in our understanding of the molecular progression of primary human cancers. Characterizing the molecular progression of a particular tumour type is critical in order to provide markers for diagnostic molecular assays. Using the appropriate marker or panel of markers would then provide information about the presence or absence of (minimal) residual cancer or unresected premalignant lesions, at this moment theoretically the best prognosticators of relapse in head and neck cancer. Point mutations in oncogenes and tumour suppressor genes, microsatellite markers, as well as tissue-specific transcripts, have all been used as markers to detect the presence of small numbers of tumour cells from solid tumours. Recent advances in the field of molecular genetics have provided extremely sensitive (RT)-PCR methods which enable the sensitive detection of tumour cells through the amplification of tumour-specific or tumour-associated (marker) nucleotide sequences in DNA or RNA. PCR-based techniques are much more sensitive in identifying cancer cells than standard techniques and, at present, various molecular markers (p53 point mutations, E48 transcripts, LOH) are available that show promise for the detection of minimal cancer in HNSCC patients, but also for the detection and grading of unresected premalignant lesions. However, the exact potential for clinical decision-making of all potential approaches has not been established yet, and necessitates prospective studies of a large number of patients with long-term follow-up. These prospective studies have to show whether minimal cancer as detected by molecular analysis is indeed a cause of locoregional or distant relapse and influences prognosis of the individual patient. Once its prognostic value has been established, molecular techniques might find acceptance in the clinic for improved staging and a more individualized treatment planning for cancer patients. In the meantime, the identification of new molecular markers and the development of new technologies is an ongoing process to provide the tools necessary for a widespread implementation of molecular techniques in clinical routine.

REFERENCES

1. Boring CC, Squires TS, Tong T. Cancer statistics. CA Cancer J Clin. 1992;42:19–38.
2. Howaldt HP, Kainz, M. Projektbericht des Zentralregisters der Deutsch-Österreichisch-Schweizerischen Arbeiteitskreises für Tumoren im Kiefer- und Gesichtsbereich, 1992.

3. Franceschi D, Gupta R, Spiro RH, Shah JP. Improved survival in the treatment of squamous carcinoma of the oral tongue. Am J Surgery. 1993;166:360–5.
4. Zarbo RJ, Crissman JD. The surgical pathology of head and neck cancer. Seminars in Oncology. 1988;15:10–19.
5. Alvi A, Johnson JT. Development of distant metastasis after treatment of advanced-stage head and neck cancer. Head & Neck. 1997;19:500–5.
6. Vikram B. Changing patterns of failure in advanced head and neck cancer. Arch Otolaryngol. 1984;110:564–5.
7. Hannahs KJ, Hooper JA, Sigler A. Nursing care of the head and neck cancer patient. In: Suen JY, Myers EN (eds) Cancer of the Head and Neck. Churchill Livingstone, New York, 1981, p. 839.
8. Callery CD, Spiro RH, Strong EW. Changing trends in the management of squamous carcinoma of the tongue. Am J Surgery. 1984;148:449–54.
9. Crile G. Excision of cancer of the head and neck – with special reference to the plan of dissection based on one hundred and thirty-two operations. J Am Med Ass. 1906;47:1780–7.
10. Brizel DM, Albers ME, Fisher SR, Scher RL, Richtsmeier WJ, Hars V *et al.* Hyperfractionated irradiation with or without concurrent chemotherapy for locally advanced head and neck. New Engl J Med. 1998;338:1798–804.
11. McGuirt WF, Johnson JT, Myers EN, Rothfield R, Wagner R. Floor of mouth carcinoma. The management of the clinically negative neck. Arch Otolaryngol Head & Neck Surg. 1995;121:278–82.
12. Petruzzelli GJ, Benefield J, Yong S. Mechanism of lymph node metastases: current concepts. Otolaryngology. Clin North Am. 1998;31:585–99.
13. Tupchong L, Scott CB, Blitzer PH, Marcial VA, Lowry LD, Jacobs JR *et al.* Randomized study of preoperative versus postoperative radiation therapy in advanced head and neck carcinoma: long-term follow-up of RTOG study 73–03. Int. J Rad Oncol. 1991;20:21–8.
14. Vokes EE, Weichselbaum RR, Lippman SM, Hong KW. Medical Progress; Head and Neck Cancer. New Engl J Med. 1993;328:184–94.
15. Harrison LB, Lee HJ, Pfister DG, Kraus DH, White C, Raben A *et al.* Long term results of primary radiotherapy with/without neck dissection for squamous cell cancer of the base of tongue. Head & Neck. 1998;20:668–73.
16. Fisher B, Fisher ER. Barrier function of lymph node to tumour cells and erythrocytes; I Normal nodes; II Effect of X-Ray/inflammation/sensitization and tumour growth. Cancer. 1967;20:1907–19.
17. Jones AS, Roland NJ, Field JK, Phillips DE. The level of cervical lymph node metastases: their prognostic relevance and relationship with head and neck squamous carcinoma primary sites. Clin Otolaryngol. 1994;19:63–9.
18. Snow GB, Annyas AA, Van Slooten EA, Bartelink H, Hart AAM. Prognostic factors of neck node metastasis. Clin Otolaryngol. 1982;7:185–92.
19. Leemans ChR, Tiwari R, Nauta JJ, Van der Waal I, Snow GB. Regional lymph node involvement and its significance in the development of distant metastases in head and neck carcinoma. Cancer. 1993;71:452–6.
20. Violaris NS, O'Neil D, Helliwell TR, Caslin AW, Roland NJ, Jones AS. Soft tissue cervical metastases of squamous carcinoma of the head and neck. Clin Otolaryngol. 1993;19:394–9.
21. Lindberg R. Distribution of cervical lymph node metastases from squamous cell carcinoma of the upper respiratory and digestive tracts. Cancer. 1972;29:1446–9.

22. Shah JP, Candela FC, Poddar AK. The patterns of cervical lymph node metastases from squamous carcinoma of the oral cavity. Cancer. 1990;66:109–13.
23. Shah JP. Patterns of cervical lymph node metastasis from squamous carcinomas of the upper aerodigestive tract. Am J Surgery. 1990;160:405–9.
24. Candela FC, Kothari K, Shah JP. Patterns of cervical node metastases from squamous carcinoma of the oropharynx and hypopharynx. Head & Neck. 1990;12:197–203.
25. Candela FC, Shah J, Jaques DP, Shah JP. Patterns of cervical node metastases from squamous carcinoma of the larynx. Arch Otolaryngol Head & Neck Surg. 1990;4:432–5.
26. Bataini JP, Bernier J, Brugere J, Jaulerry Ch, Picco Ch, Brunin F. Natural history of neck disease in patients with squamous cell carcinoma of oropharynx and pharyngolarynx. Radiother Oncol. 1985;3:245–55.
27. Lindberg RD. Distribution of cervical lymph node metastases from squamous cell carcinoma of the upper respiratory and digestive tracts. Cancer. 1972;29:1446–9.
28. Kinsey DL, James AG, Bonta JA. A study of metastatic carcinoma of the neck. Ann Surg. 1985;147: 366–74.
29. Byers RM, Wolf PF, Ballantyne AJ. Rationale for elective modified neck dissection. Head & Neck. Surg. 1988;3:160–7.
30. Byers RM, Weber RS, Andrews T, McGill D, Kare R, Wolf P. Frequency and therapeutic implications of 'skip metastases' in the neck from squamous carcinoma of the oral tongue. Head & Neck. 1997;19:14–19.
31. Dennington ML, Carter DR, Meijers AD. Distant metastases in head and neck carcinoma. Laryngoscope. 1980;90:196–201.
32. Nishijima W, Takooda S, Tokita N, Takayama S, Sakura M. Analyses of distant metastases in squamous cell carcinoma of the head and neck and lesions above the clavicle at autopsy. Arch Otolaryngol Head & Neck. Surgery. 1993;119:65–8.
33. Zbären P, Lehmann W. Frequency and sites of distant metastases in head and neck squamous cell carcinoma. An analysis of 101 cases at autopsy. Arch Otolaryng Head & Neck Surg. 1987;113:762–4.
34. Spiro RH. The management of neck nodes in head and neck cancer: a surgeon's view. Bulletin NY Acad Med. 1985;61:629–37.
35. Vernham GA, Crowther JA. Head and neck carcinoma – stage at presentation. Clin Otolaryngol. 1994;19:120–4.
36. Cooper JS, Pajak TF, Rubin P, Tupchong L, Brady LW, Leibel SA *et al.* Second malignancies in patients who have head and neck cancer: incidence, effect on survival and implications based on the RTOG experience. Int J Radiat Oncol. 1989; 17:449–56.
37. Licciardello JT, Spitz MR, Hong WK. Multiple primary cancer in patients with cancer of the head and neck: second cancer of the head and neck, esophagus, and lung. Int J Radiat Oncol. 1989;17:467–76.
38. Schaart LH, Ozsahin M, Zhang GN, Touboul E, De-Vataire F, Andolenko P *et al.* Synchronous and metachronous head and neck carcinomas. Cancer. 1994;74:1933–8.
39. Warren S, Gates O. Multiple primary malignant tumours: a survey of the literature and a statistical study. Am J Cancer. 1932;16:1358–414.
40. Hong WK, Lippman SM, Itri LM, Karp DD, Lee JS, Byers RM *et al.* Prevention of second primary tumours with isotretinoin in squamous-cell carcinoma of the head and neck. New Engl J Med. 1990;323:795–801.

41. Bedi GC, Westra WH, Gabrielson E, Koch W, Sidransky D. Multiple head and neck tumours: evidence for a common clonal origin. Cancer Res. 1996;56:2484–7.
42. Leong PP, Rezai B, Koch WM, Reed A, Eisele D, Lee DJ *et al.* Distinguishing second primary tumours from lung metastases in patients with head and neck squamous cell carcinoma. J Natl Cancer Inst. 1998;90: 972–7.
43. Slaughter DP, Southwick HW, Smejkal W. Field cancerisation in oral stratified squamous epithelium: clinical implication of multicentric orgin. Cancer. 1953;6:963–8.
44. Cloos J, Braakhuis BJM, Steen I, Copper MP, de Vries N, Nauta JJP, Snow GB. Increased mutagen sensitivity in head-and-neck squamous-cell carcinoma patients, particularly those with multiple primary tumours. Int J Cancer. 1994;56:816–19.
45. Cloos J, Spitz MR, Schantz SP, Hsu TC, Zhang Z, Tobi H *et al.* Genetic susceptibility to head and neck squamous cell carcinoma. J Natl Cancer Inst. 1996;88:530–5.
46. Cloos J, Nieuwenhuis EJC, Boomsma DI, Kuik DJ, van der Sterre MLT, Arwert F *et al.* Inherited susceptibility to bleomycin-induced chromatid breaks in cultured peripheral blood lymphocytes. J Natl Cancer Inst. 1999;91:1125–30.
47. Van Zandwijk N, Dalesio O, Pastorino U, De Vries N, Van Tinteren, H. EUROSCAN, a randomized trial of vitamin A and N-acetylcysteine in patients with head and neck cancer or lung cancer. J Natl Cancer Inst. 2000;92:977–86.
48. Lee JJ, Hong WK, Hittelman WN, Mao L, Lotan R, Shin DM *et al.* Predicting cancer development in oral leukoplakia: Ten years of translational research. Clin Cancer Res. 2000;6:1702–10.
49. Fearon ER, Vogelstein B. A genetic model for colorectal tumourigenesis. Cell. 1990;61:759–67.
50. Cairns P, Sidransky D. Molecular methods for the diagnosis of cancer. Biochem Biophys Acta. 1999;1423:C11–18.
51. Sidransky D. Nucleic acid-based methods for the detection of cancer. Science. 1997;278:1054–9.
52. Weber JL, May PE. Abundant class of human DNA polymorphisms which can be typed using the polymerase chain reaction. Am J Hum Genet. 1989;44:388–96.
53. Califano J, van der Riet P, Westra W, Nawroz H, Clayman G, Piantadosi S *et al.* Genetic progression model for head and neck cancer: implications for field cancerization. Cancer Res. 1996;56:2488–92.
54. Hollstein M, Sidransky D, Vogelstein, B, Harris CC. P53 mutations in human cancers. Science. 1991;253:49–53.
55. Greenblatt MS, Bennett WP, Hollstein M, Harris CC. Mutations in the p53 tumour suppressor gene: clues to cancer etiology and molecular pathogenesis. Cancer Res. 1994;54:4855–78.
56. Van Houten VMM, Snijders PJF, Van den Brekel MWM, Meijer CJML, Van Leeuwen B, Smeele LE *et al.* Biological evidence that human papillomaviruses are etiologically involved in a subgroup of head and neck squamous cell carcinomas. Int J Cancer. 2001;93:232–5.
57. Sidransky D, Von Eschenbach A, Tsai YC, Jones P, Summerhayes I, Marshall F *et al.* Identification of p53 gene mutations in bladder cancers and urine samples. Science. 1991;252:706–9.
58. Steiner G, Schoenberg MP, Linn JF, Mao L, Sidransky D. Detection of bladder cancer recurrence by microsatellite analysis of urine. Nature Med. 1997;3:621–4.
59. Brennan JA, Mao L, Hruban RH, Boyle JO, Eby YJ, Koch WM *et al.* Molecular assessment of histopathological staging in squamous-cell carcinoma of the head and neck. N Engl J Med. 1995;332:429–35.

60. Takeda S, Ichii S, Nakamura Y. Detection of K-ras mutation in sputum by mutant-allele-specific amplification (MASA). Hum Mutation. 1993;2:112–17.
61. Landegren U, Kaiser R, Sanders J, Hood L. A ligase-mediated gene detection technique. Science. 1988;241:1077–80.
62. Somers VA, Moerkerk PT, Murtagh JJ. Jr, Thunnessen FB. A rapid, reliable method for detection of known point mutations: POINT-EXACCT. Nucl Acids Res. 1994;22:4840–1.
63. Kahn SM, Jiang W, Culbertson TA, Weinstein IB, Williams GM, Tomita N *et al.* Rapid and sensitive non-radioactive detection of mutant K-ras genes via enriched PCR amplification. Oncogene. 1991;6:1079–83.
64. Levi S, Urbanoispizua A, Gill R, Thomas DM, Gilbertson J, Foster C *et al.* Multiple K-ras codon-12 mutations in cholangiocarcinomas demonstrated with a sensitive polymerase chain-reaction technique. Cancer Res. 1991;51:3497–502.
65. Behn M, Qun S, Pankow W, Havemann K, Schuermann M. Frequent detection of RAS and p53 mutations in brush cytology samples from lung cancer patients by a restriction fragment length polymorphism-based 'Enriched PCR' technique. Clin Cancer Res. 1998;4:361–71.
66. Ward R, Hawkins N, O'Grady R, Sheehan C, O'Connor T, Impey H *et al.* Restriction endonuclease-mediated selective polymerase chain reaction – a novel assay for the detection of K-ras mutations in clinical samples. Am J Pathol. 1998;153:373–9.
67. Vogelstein B, Kinzler KW. Digital PCR. Proc Natl Acad Sci USA. 1999;96:9236–41.
68. Ahrendt SA, Halachmi S, Chow JT, Wu L, Halachmi N, Yang SC *et al.* Rapid p53 sequence analysis in primary lung cancer using an oligonucleotide probe array. Proc Natl Acad Sci USA. 1999;96:7382–7.
69. Fu DJ, Tang K, Braun A, Reuter D, Darnhoferdemar B, Little DP *et al.* Sequencing exons 5 to 8 of the p53 gene by MALDI-TOF mass spectrometry. Nature Biotech. 1998;16:381–4.
70. Williams C, Ponten F, Moberg C, Soderkvist P, Uhlen M, Ponten J *et al.* A high frequency of sequence alterations is due to formalin fixation of archival specimens. Am J Pathol. 1999;155:1467–71.
71. Brennan JA, Sidransky D. Molecular staging of head and neck squamous carcinoma. Cancer Metast Rev. 1996;15:3–10.
72. Sakai E, Tsuchida,N. Most human squamous cell carcinomas in the oral cavity contain mutated p53 tumour-suppressor genes. Oncogene. 1992;7:927–33.
73. Burns JE, McFarlane R, Clark LJ, Mitchell R, Robertson G, Soutar D *et al.* Maintenance of identical p53 mutations throughout progression of squamous cell carcinomas of the tongue. Eur J Cancer Part B, Oral Oncology. 1994; 30B:335–7.
74. Tjebbes GWA, Van der Straat FGJL, Tilanus MGJ, Hordijk GJ, Slootweg PJ. P53 tumour suppressor gene as a clonal marker in head and neck squamous cell carcinoma: p53 mutations in primary tumour and matched lymph node metastases. Oral Oncology. 1999;35:384–9.
75. Zariwala M, Schmid S, Pfaltz M, Ohgaki H, Kleihues P, Schafer R. P53 gene mutations in oropharyngeal carcinomas: a comparison of solitary and multiple primary tumours and lymph-node metastases. Int J Cancer. 1994;56:807–11.
76. Ahomadegbe JC, Barrois M, Fogel S, Le Bihan ML, Douc-Rasy S, Duvillard P *et al.* High incidence of p53 alterations (mutation, deletion, overexpression) in head and neck primary tumours and metastases, absence of correlation with clinical outcome. Frequent protein overexpression in normal epithelium and in early non-invasive lesions. Oncogene. 1995;10:1217–27.

77. Kropveld A, Van Mansfeld AD, Nabben N, Hordijk GJ, Slootweg PJ. Discordance of p53 status in matched primary tumours and metastases in head and neck squamous cell carcinoma patients. Eur J Cancer Part B, Oral Oncology. 1996; 32B:388–93.
78. Tabor MP, Van Houten VMM, Kummer JA, Vosjan MJWD, Vlasblom R, Snow GB, Leemans ChR *et al.* Discordance of genetic alterations between primary head and neck tumours and corresponding metastases associated with mutational status of the TP53 gene. Genes Chrom Cancer. 2001;33:168–77.
79. Kropveld A, Rozemuller EH, Leppers FGJ, Scheidel KC, de Weger RA, Koole R *et al.* Sequencing analysis of RNA and DNA of exons 1 through 11 shows p53 gene alterations to be present in almost 100% of head and neck squamous cell cancers. Lab Invest. 1999;79:347–53.
80. Van Houten V, Denkers F, Van Dijk M, Van den Brekel M, Brakenhoff, R. Labeling efficiency of oligonucleotides by T4 polynucleotide kinase depends on 5′-nucleotide. Anal Biochem. 1998;265:386–9.
81. Van Houten VMM, Tabor MP, Van den Brekel MWM, Denkers F, Wishaupt RGA, Kummer JA *et al.* Molecular assays for the diagnosis of minimal residual head and neck cancer: methods, reliability, pitfalls and solutions. Clin Cancer Res. 2000;6:3803–16.
82. Nawroz H, Koch W, Anker P, Stroun M, Sidransky D. Microsatellite alterations in serum DNA of head and neck cancer patients. Nature Med. 1996;2:1035–7.
83. Jahr S, Hentze H, Englisch S, Hardt D, Fackelmayer FO, Hesch RD, Knippers R. DNA fragments in the blood plasma of cancer patients: quantitations and evidence for their origin from apoptotic and necrotic cells. Cancer Res. 2001;61: 1659–65.
84. Tindall KR, Kunkel TA. Fidelity of DNA synthesis by the Thermus aquaticus DNA polymerase. Biochemistry. 1988;27:6008–13.
85. Saiki RK, Gelfand DH, Stoffel S, Scharf SJ, Higuchi R, Horn GT *et al.* Primer-directed enzymatic amplification of DNA with a thermostable DNA polymerase. Science. 1988;239:487–91.
86. Nees M, Homann N, Discher H, Andl T, Enders C, Herold-Mende C *et al.* Expression of mutated p53 occurs in tumour-distant epithelia of head and neck cancer patients: a possible molecular basis for the development of multiple tumours. Cancer Res. 1993;53:4189–96.
87. Cruz IB, Snijders PJF, Meijer CJLM, Braakhuis BJM, Snow GB, Walboomers JMM *et al.* P53 expression above the basal cell layer in oral mucosa is an early event of malignant transformation and has predictive value for developing oral squamous cell carcinoma. J Pathol. 1998;184:360–8.
88. Knudson AG Jr. Mutation and cancer: statistical study of retinoblastoma. Proc Natl Acad Sci USA. 1971;68:820–3.
89. Boland CR, Thibodeau SN, Hamilton SR, Sidransky D, Eshleman JR, Burt RW *et al.* National Cancer Institute Workshop on Microsatellite Instability for Cancer Detection and Familial Predisposition: development of international criteria for the determination of microsatellite instability in colorectal cancer. Cancer Res. 1998;58:5248–57.
90. Aaltonen LA, Peltomaki P, Leach FS, Sistonen P, Pylkkanen L, Mecklin JP *et al.* Clues to the pathogenesis of familial colorectal cancer. Science. 1993;260:812–16.
91. Vogelstein B. Lessons from hereditary colorectal cancer. Cell. 1996;87:159–70.
92. Tabor MP, Brakenhoff RH, Van Houten VMM, Kummer JA, Snel MHJ, Snijders PJF *et al.* Persistence of genetically altered fields in head and neck cancer patients: biological and clinical implications. Clin Cancer Res. 2001;7:1523–32.

93. Braakhuis BJM, Tabor MP, Leemans ChR, Van der Waal I, Snow GB, Brakenhoff, RH. Second primary tumours and field cancerization in oral and oropharyngeal cancer: molecular techniques provide new insights and definitions. Head & Neck. 2002; 24:198–206.
94. Ashworth TA. A case of cancer in which cells similar to those in the tumours were seen in the blood after death. Australian Med J. 1869;14:146.
95. Lindemann F, Schlimok G, Dirschedl P, Witte J, Riethmüller G. Prognostic significance of micrometastatic tumour cells in bone marrow of colorectal cancer. Lancet. 1992;340:685–9.
96. Pantel K, Izbicki J, Passlick B, Angstwurm M, Häussinger K, Thetter O *et al.* Frequency and prognostic significance of isolated tumour cells in bone marrow of patients with non-small-cell lung cancer without overt metastases. Lancet. 1996;347:649–53.
97. Braun S, Pantel K, Muller P, Janni W, Hepp F, Kentenich CRM *et al.* Cytokeratin-positive cells in the bone marrow and survival of patients with stage I, II, or III breast cancer. New Engl J Med. 2000;342:525–33.
98. Wollenberg B, Ollesch A, Maag K, Funke I, Wilmes E. Mikrometastasen im knockenmark von patienten mit karzinomen des kopf-hals-bereiches. Laryngo Rhino Otol. 1994;73:88–93.
99. Gath H, Brakenhoff RH. Minimal residual disease in head and neck cancer. Cancer Metas Rev. 1999;18:109–26.
100. Brakenhoff, RH, Stroomer JGW, Ten Brink C, De Bree R, Weima SM, Snow GB *et al.* Sensitive detection of squamous cells in bone marrow and blood of head and neck cancer patients by E48 reverse transcriptase polymerase chain reaction. Clin Cancer Res. 1999;5:725–32.
101. Nieuwenhuis EJC, Castelijns JA, Pijpers R, Van den Brekel MWM, Brakenhoff RH, Van der Waal I *et al.* Wait and see policy for the N0 neck in early stage oral and oropharyngeal SCC using ultrasound guided cytology: is there a role for identification of the sentinel node. Head & Neck. 2002;24:282–9.
102. Nieuwenhuis EJC, Jaspers EHJ, Castelijns JA, Bakker B, Wishaupt RGA, Denkers F, Leemans ChR, Snow GB, Brakenhoff RH. Quantitative molecular detection of minimal residual head and neck cancer in lymph node aspirates. Clin Cancer Res. 2003;9:755–61.

Chapter 3

DETECTION AND CHARACTERISATION OF OCCULT METASTATIC CELLS IN BONE MARROW OF BREAST CANCER PATIENTS: IMPLICATIONS FOR ADJUVANT THERAPY

Stephan Braun[1], Volkmar Müller[2,3], Klaus Pantel[2]

[1]Universitätsklinik für Frauenheilkunde, Leopold-Franzens-Universität, Anichstrasse 35, A-6020 Innsbruck, Austria; [2]Institut für Tumorbiologie, Universitätsklinikum Eppendorf, Martinistrasse 52, D-20246 Hamburg, Germany; [3]Klinik für Frauenheilkunde, Universitätsklinikum Eppendorf, Martinistrasse 52, D-20246 Hamburg, Germany

Abstract

The early and clinically occult spread of viable tumour cells to the organism is becoming acknowledged as a hallmark in cancer progression, since abundant clinical and experimental data suggest that these cells are precursors of subsequent distant relapse. Prospective clinical studies have shown that the presence of such immunostained cells in bone marrow is prognostically relevant with regard to relapse-free and overall survival of breast cancer patients. As current treatment strategies have not resulted in a substantial improvement of breast cancer mortality rates so far, it is noteworthy to consider the intriguing options of immunocytochemical screening of bone marrow aspirates for occult metastatic cells. Besides improved tumour staging, such screening offers opportunities for guiding patient stratification for adjuvant therapy trials, monitoring response to adjuvant therapies, which, at present, can only be assessed retrospectively after an extended period of clinical follow-up, or for specifically targeting tumour-biological therapies against disseminated tumour cells.

1. INTRODUCTION

Occult dissemination of tumour cells in patients with operable breast cancer may be a crucial step in carcinogenesis and subsequent metastasis formation, yet conventional tumour staging usually does not reveal it. To identify individual tumour cells that have successfully escaped from the primary tumour and invaded secondary organs several research groups established sensitive immunocytochemical and molecular assays (1). Because of its easy accessibility and physiological absence of epithelial cells, bone marrow plays a prominent role as determinant for micrometastatic organ involvement (2–4). In breast cancer, bone also represents a relevant site of distant metastasis suggesting that bone marrow is a relevant site

K. Pantel (ed.), Micrometastasis, 47–65.

for the search of early dissemination of metastatic cells. In consequence, the development of antibodies to epithelial differentiation antigens, such as cytokeratins, as major constituents of the epithelial cytoskeleton, and tumour-associated cell membrane glycoproteins, enabled diagnosis of disseminated tumour cells as early as at primary diagnosis (2, 5).

Compared to the well-documented prognostic significance of isolated tumour cells disseminated to bone marrow, their biological characteristics remain poorly understood. This lack of knowledge requires an explanation, particularly for patients with micrometastatic bone marrow involvement who have not developed manifest (bone) metastasis during observation after surgery. It is therefore conceivable that differential biological properties of disseminated tumour cells in bone marrow exist. Individual characteristics of the respective tumour cells influence their differential homing and outgrowth of metastases. Thus, disseminated tumour cells may not necessarily have the potential to form clinically detectable metastases in this particular environment, but may rather remain dormant for years. Support for the concept of dormancy is also derived from the clinical observation that distant metastases can manifest themselves as late as 10 years after the excision of a primary tumour (6).

The emerging data supporting the prognostic relevance of this phenomenon (7) point out that appropriate therapeutic approaches directed against dormant micrometastatic cancer cells need to be evolved urgently. It is known from the clinical practice that both loco-regional and distant tumour recurrences occurred in patients treated with curative intent, e.g., complete tumour resection (R0) in patients without lymph node (N0) and distant metastases (M0). This is also true in cases where systemic cytotoxic chemotherapy was applied, which pointed to the existence of at least some resistant tumour cells. Although various mechanisms may contribute to this apparent chemo-resistance, the latter assumption could be supported by the absence of proliferation-associated markers on disseminated tumour cells in bone marrow (8). In this view cell cycle independent treatment strategies, such as antibody-based immunotherapy, which have been recently shown to be active in breast cancer (9, 10), might gain increased interest for the design of future clinical trials. The present review focuses on the prognostic relevance and characterisation of occult metastatic cells in bone marrow of breast cancer patients and the implications of this knowledge for adjuvant therapy.

2. PROGNOSTIC RELEVANCE OF OCCULT METASTATIC CELLS

Before elucidating the implications of occult metastatic cells for systemic cancer treatment, it needs to be clarified how the presence of such cells contributes to a clinically relevant stratification for specific therapy. From a clinical point of view, it also needs to be discussed which of the investigated body compartments – including bone marrow (BM), peripheral blood (PB), and lymph nodes (LN) – provide the most reliable prognostic estimation.

BM has so far played a prominent role as an indicator organ of occult tumour cell dissemination. It is easily accessible for the clinician by aspiration, tumour cells found in this compartment are likely to have actively invaded the parenchyma, and bone represents a clinically relevant site for distant metastasis in breast cancer and other solid tumours. Our own experience shows that repeated BM aspiration is feasible and associated with extremely low patient morbidity (11).

PB provides the advantage that every clinician is familiar with blood tests, which are quickly done and can be deliberately repeated. However, the clinical significance of this approach is seriously questioned by the fact that barely 1 out of 10^4 tumour cells is able to survive shear stress and trapping in the capillary bed, escape the host's immune defence mechanisms, and subsequently evade into a secondary organ with appropriate microenvironment.

Regional LNs are of particular interest since examination of LN involvement is implemented in and validated for all major tumour risk classification systems. With respect to therapy, the major disadvantage of this compartment is that, once LNs are resected together with the primary cancer for tumour staging, no monitoring during adjuvant therapy is feasible – in contrast to the two other compartments, BM and PB.

Finally, an important issue for treatment evaluation is the quantification of any therapeutic effect. In order to be able to determine a quantifiable difference of tumour cells in pre- and post-therapeutic samples, it is mandatory that the number of tumour cells can be reliably related to the background of non-tumour (e.g., BM) cells. This is only feasible in cytospin preparations, which allow a reliable transfer of a defined number of cells to the analysed slide (3, 12). In contrast, the number of cells in BM smears and sections of BM biopsies cannot be reliably determined and may vary from preparation to preparation, which inevitably leads to poor precision in terms of cellular quantification and, hence, reproducibility.

2.1 Bone Marrow

Although the search for occult metastatic cells was initiated in patients with breast cancer about 20 years ago (13–15), studies in patients with colorectal, gastric, pancreatic, oesophageal, or non-small lung cell cancer increased the interest in minimal residual disease in solid tumours among basic scientists and clinicians. It is perhaps of some irony that the clinical relevance of minimal residual disease in breast cancer, a disease known for its preference for bone meta-stases, is still under discussion due to discrepancies between some studies (16). The currently available data on the prognostic impact of occult metastatic cells is summarised in Table 1. While numerous studies confirmed the prognostic influence of occult metastatic cells on relapse-free and overall survival in patients with breast cancer (4, 17–24), some studies failed to do so (25–32).

Thus, a large-scale study using an immunoassay with proven sensitivity and specificity was warranted in order to demonstrate whether or not a positive immunocytochemical finding indeed reflects presence of tumour cells and

Table 1. Occult metastatic cancer cells in bone marrow of breast cancer patients

References	Marker*	Technique	# Pts.	Detection Rate	Prognostic Value
Porro *et al.* (32)	Mucin	ICC	159	16%	none
Salvadori *et al.* (31)	Mucin	ICC	121	17%	none
Mathieu *et al.* (30)	Mucin/CK	ICC	93	1%	none
Courtemanche *et al.* (28)	Mucin	ICC	50	8%	none
Landys *et al.* (21)	CK	ICC	128	19%	DFS†, OS†
Singletary *et al.* (29)	Mucin/CK	ICC	71	38%	none
Cote *et al.* (24)	Mucin/CK	ICC	49	37%	DFS, OS
Harbeck *et al.* (23)	Mucin/CK	ICC	100	38%	DFS†, OS†
Diel *et al.* (22)	Mucin	ICC	727	43%	DFS†, OS†
Funke *et al.* (27)	CK18	ICC	234	38%	n.d.
Untch *et al.* (25)	CK18	ICC	581	28%	none
Mansi *et al.* (20)	Mucin	ICC	350	25%	DFS, OS
Gebauer *et al.* (17)	Mucin	ICC	393	42%	DFS†, OS
Braun *et al.* (4)	CK	ICC	552	36%	DDFS†, OS†
Gerber *et al.* (19)	CK	ICC	484	31%	DFS†, OS†
Braun *et al.* (18)	CK	ICC	150	29%	DDFS†, OS†
Datta *et al.* (34)	CK19	RT-PCR	34	26%	DFS
Fields *et al.* (35)	CK19	RT-PCR	83	71%	DFS
Vannucchi *et al.* (36)	CK19	RT-PCR	33	48%	DFS
Slade *et al.* (37)	CK19	RT-PCR	23	61%	none

Notes: *Abbreviations: CK, cytokeratin; DFS, disease-free survival; DDFS, distant disease-free survival; ICC = immunocytochemistry; OS, overall survival; RT-PCR = reverse-transcriptase polymerase-chain reaction. †Prognostic value supported by multivariate analysis.

impacts on patient outcome. To dispel the prevailing doubts as to the accuracy of methodology and size of study populations, we performed a prospectively planned study on 552 newly diagnosed patients with Stage I–III breast cancer, using a validated immunoassay (3, 33) that rendered reproducible results at both centres of the study (4). In this study, we found that the presence of occult metastatic cells in BM was associated with the occurrence of clinically overt distant metastasis and death from cancer-related causes. In addition, in clinically relevant subgroups, the presence of occult metastatic cells distinguished between marrow-negative patients with fairly good prognosis and marrow-positive patients with worse outcome in respect to disease-free and overall survival. Particularly, as verified by multivariate regression analyses, the presence of occult metastatic cells in BM predicted poor prognosis independently of LN metastases (4).

2.2 Peripheral Blood

In contrast to BM, only a few studies on PB screening (37–39) have been so far conducted (Table 2). Utilisation of PB as an indicator organ of occult metastatic cells is an extremely interesting issue for screening and monitoring. The clinical significance of circulating tumour cells in PB is, however, seriously questioned by the fact that barely 1 out of 10^4 tumour cells is able to survive shear stress and trapping in the capillary bed, escape the host's immune defence mechanisms, and subsequently evade into a secondary organ with an appropriate microenvironment. The currently available data do not provide any evidence of the prognostic impact of positive findings.

2.3 Lymph Nodes

Regional LNs are examined regularly in patients with breast cancer since LN involvement is implemented in all major tumour risk classification systems. Now the question has to be raised whether the LN involvement correlates with the presence of occult metastatic cells in other body compartments, such as BM, and how it can be modified for its use in patients with node-negative breast cancer.

So far, numerous studies (Table 2) have demonstrated that the presence of immunocytochemically identified LN micrometastases, in breast cancer patients presumed to be node-negative after conventional histology, indicate poor patient outcome (e.g., 19, 40, 41, 42, 44, 45). Among these patients with node-negative disease approximately one-third will recur with distant disease within five years after surgery (2, 48). Already in the 1970s it was shown in animal models (49)

Table 2. Occult metastatic cancer cells in peripheral blood or lymph nodes of breast cancer patients

References	Marker*	Technique	# Pts.	Detection Rate	Prognostic Value
Peripheral blood					
Mapara *et al.* (38)	CK/EGFR	RT-PCR	21	81%	none
Slade *et al.* (37)	CK19	RT-PCR	37	54%	none
Zach *et al.* (39)	hMAM	RT-PCR	114	25%	none
Lymph nodes					
Bettelheim *et al.* (40)	–	H&E	927	9%	DFS†, OS†
De Mascarel *et al.* (41)	–	H&E	1,680	7%	DFS, OS
Cote *et al.* (45)	–	H&E	736	7%	DFS†, OS†
Bussolati *et al.* (42)	Mucin/CK	IHC	50	23%	DFS
De Mascarel *et al.* (41)	CK	IHC	129	10%	DFS
Nasser *et al.* (43)	CK	IHC	159	31%	none
McGuckin *et al.* (44)	Mucin/CK	IHC	208	25%	DFS†
Cote *et al.* (45)	CK	IHC	736	20%	none
Gerber *et al.* (19)	CK	IHC	484	11%	DFS†
Braun *et al.* (18)	CK	IHC	150	9%	none
Noguchi *et al.* (46)	Mucin-1	RT-PCR	15	30%	none
Schönfeld *et al.* (47)	CK19	RT-PCR	75	31%	none

Notes: *Abbreviations: CK, cytokeratin; DFS, disease-free survival; DDFS, distant disease-free survival; EGFR = epithelial growth factor receptor; H&E = hematoxylin and eosin staining; hMAM = human mammaglobin; IHC = immunohistochemistry; OS, overall survival; RT-PCR = reverse-transcriptase polymerase-chain reaction. †Prognostic value supported by multivariate analysis.

that the presence of LN metastases does not necessarily correlate with the presence of distant metastases. In a first study comparing directly the presence of LN micrometastases with that of BM micrometastases in presumed node-negative patients, we found a prevalence of 9% and 29%, respectively (18). Interestingly, a coincidence of isolated tumour cells in BM and LNs was found in only two patients (1.3%). Reduced distant disease-free and overall survival were only associated with a positive BM finding ($P = 0.039$ and $P = 0.014$, respectively) but not with LN micrometastases. These results were essentially confirmed in a second study on 484 patients, with a prevalence of 11% LN and 31% BM micrometastases, and a coincidence of LN and BM micrometastases in 5% using antibodies directed against CK8, CK18, and CK19 (19).

3. BIOLOGICAL CHARACTERISTICS OF OCCULT METASTATIC CELLS

The convincing data on prognostic and predictive value of isolated tumour cells disseminated to BM inaugurated the search for biological characteristics of the primary tumour that might be decisive for early dissemination. Applying immunocytochemical double labelling methods micrometastases can be identified and characterised directly (8, 50–53). Related to the malignant potential of CK-positive cells, a variety of tumour-associated characteristics have been identified, applying these methods to elucidate among others the expression of urokinase-plasminogen activator (uPA)-receptor, over-expression of the erb-B2 oncogene, and deficient expression of MCH class I molecules (Table 3).

The evaluation of possible correlation between the phenotype of primary breast carcinomas and the presence of tumour cells may be another step towards the detection of structures that support the onset of micrometastatic spread. Two research groups were recently able to show significant correlation between tumour angiogenesis and BM micrometastases in breast and gastric cancer (54, 55). According to McCulloch *et al.*, there is an association between tumour angiogenesis and tumour cell shedding into effluent venous blood during breast cancer surgery (56, 57). Ménard *et al.* revealed that the expression of the 67-kDa laminin receptor on primary breast cancer cells may support tumour cell dissemination into LN and BM (58, 59).

3.1 Proliferation-Associated Antigens

In view of the similar rates of disseminated tumour cells detected throughout different tumour entities, the capacity of these cells to home in BM appears to be similar (51). In contrast, the potential of these tumour cells to outgrow in this new compartment seems to differ considerably.

The proliferation markers Ki-67 antigen, which can be found in all phases of the cell cycle except G0 and early G1 (60), and p120 antigen, present during early G1 with another peak in S phase (61), have been used to determine the rate of proliferating metastatic tumour cells in BM (Table 3). In BM, only one of 33 patients with Ki-67-positive/CK-positive cells was identified. While CK-positive cells revealed p120 antigen expression in 10 (28%) of 36 cases, less than 10% of CK-positive cells per specimen were found to be double p120-positive/CK-positive cells. Consequently, the majority of disseminated tumour cells appeared to be non-cycling and rest in G0 phase of the cell cycle.

The reduced proliferative activity observed in micrometastatic tumour cells at this early stage of dissemination is consistent with the well-known phenomenon of tumour cell dormancy. This phenomenon may be explained by experimental data showing that the acquisition of at least some characteristics of metastatic behaviour can occur prior to attainment of the unrestrained growth observed in fully developed tumours (62, 63). Thus, tumour cells which have undertaken the first steps in the metastatic cascade may develop their full growth

Table 3. Phenotype of disseminated cytokeratin-positive tumour cells in bone marrow

Markers	Tumour Origin	No. of Patients with Marker +/CK + Cells	(%)*
MHC class I antigen†	Breast	10/26	(38)
	Colorectum	12/17	(71)
	Stomach	8/11	(73)
Proliferation-associated protein			
Ki-67	Breast	1/12	(8)
	Colorectum	0/13	
	Stomach	0/8	
p120	Breast	1/11	(9)
	Colorectum	5/12	(28)
	Stomach	4/13	(28)
Adhesion molecule			
EpCAM† (17-1A)	Breast	23/31	(74)
Plakoglobin	Colorcctum	8/25	(32)
Growth factor receptors			
EGF-R†	Breast	10/37	(27)
	Colorectum	4/15	(26)
HER2	Breast	48/71	(68)
	Colorectum/Stomach	14/50	(28)
Transferrin-receptor	Breast	17/59	(29)
	Colorectum	7/17	(41)
$Lewis^Y$	Breast	11/14	(79)
Mucin-1	Breast	11/14	(79)
Protease uPA receptor†	Stomach	20/44	(45)
p53 tumour suppressor protein	Colorectum	4/63	(3)

Notes: *From (2, 3, 50, 52, 53, 65–67). †Abbreviations: EGF-R = epithelial growth factor receptor; EpCAM = epithelial cell adhesion molecule; MHC = major histocompatibility complex; uPA = urokinase-type plasminogen activator.

potential only years later (64). Therefore, the importance of defining markers that predict the transition from a dormant into a proliferative state is obvious.

3.2 Tumour Suppressor Genes

Several point mutations in the p53 gene lead to the expression of a stabilised mutant protein (68). Accumulation of p53 protein (TP53) became thus a marker of malignant disease in diagnostic cytopathology (69). We hence investigated the presence of such accumulation in disseminated tumour cells using double marker analysis (Table 3). Surprisingly, co-expression of TP53 was only found in 4 (3%) of 63 patients examined and was entirely absent in another series applying further epithelial markers for the detection of tumour cells, such as monoclonal antibodies to cytokeratin-19 and to an epitope shared by various cytokeratin molecules (65). According to our findings, immunodetection of TP53 appeared of little value for the identification of individual micrometastatic carcinoma cells in BM. The fact that TP53 levels have been measured only at a low frequency in these cells appears not to confirm the assumption that protein-stabilising mutations in the p53 gene provide a selective advantage for early tumour cell dissemination.

3.3 Over-Expression of erb-B2 Oncogene

Among specific receptors that may promote the outgrowth of tumour cells to manifest in BM metastases, epithelial growth factor (EGF) and transferrin, which were expressed on about 30% of CK-positive cells, may play an important role (66). Previous studies pointed out that gene amplification and over-expression of erb-B2, the oncogene encoded growth factor receptor homologue of the EGF-R, are associated with a more aggressive growth in human breast cancer (70–74). Immunodetection of $p185^{erb\text{-}B2}$ by antibodies has been shown to be correlated with over-expression of the oncoprotein (75). Typing CK-positive aspirates for $p185^{erb\text{-}B2}$ over-expression, we assessed an increased rate of $p185^{erb\text{-}B2}$ protein expression (60% on micrometastatic cells vs. 25% on primary tumours) and analysed its prognostic role (76) for occult tumour cells in BM (Table 3).

As shown by recent *in vitro* data, expression of $p185^{erb\text{-}B2}$ in human cells can induce a change in the homotypic epithelial adhesion interactions via down-regulation of E-cadherin expression (77). Accordingly, it is not surprising that $p185^{erb\text{-}B2}$-positive micrometastatic cells may have been positively selected from a small metastatic subpopulation within the primary tumour by suppressing the metastasis-suppressor function of E-cadherin. In consequence, $p185^{erb\text{-}B2}$ might be regarded as a marker for dissemination. From the increased incidence of $p185^{erb\text{-}B2}$ expression on metastatic tumour cells found in advanced-stage patients it can be concluded that such expression may as well support the survival and/or outgrowth of these cells in the BM environment. Therefore it may be of interest whether proteins claimed to act as natural ligands for the $p185^{erb\text{-}B2}$ receptor (78–80) are expressed in CK-positive cells or BM cells.

In BM tumour cells of breast cancer patients significant higher incidences of p185^{erb-B2} were measured compared to patients with gastrointestinal cancer (8) which in contrast to breast cancer is known for rarer manifestation of overt bone metastases. In addition, distinctly higher incidences of p185^{erb-B2} expression (60–70%) have been found in metastatic BM cells compared to primary tumours (25%). Therefore, p185^{erb-B2} over-expression might be a positive selection criterion for disseminated tumour cells (8). All of the breast cancer patients with manifest distant metastases (M1) investigated exhibited p185^{erb-B2} on CK-positive cells compared to about 50% of the patients with loco-regional disease (M0) (8). Recently, Brandt *et al.* suggested that blood-borne p185^{erb-B2}-positive/CK-positive clustered cells might be precursors of distant (micro-) metastases (81). These findings might explain the apparent success of antibody-therapy directed against p185^{erb-B2}-expressing cancer cells in patients with metastatic breast cancer receiving additional chemotherapy (9, 10).

3.4 Proteins Relevant to the Immunological Anti-Tumour Defence

The survival of isolated tumour cells in BM without being killed by the immune system (82) could be explained with an inability of immune effector cells to recognise these cells and/or an anergic state of the effector cells. In order to analyse how CK-positive cells escape recognition by immune effector cells, we applied our double marker assay to phenotype CK-positive cells for the expression of HLA class I molecules (53, 83). In total, 25 (46%) of 54 patients yielded CK-positive cells that lacked a detectable expression of HLA class I molecules (Table 3). In breast cancer patients, 65% HLA-negative carcinoma cells in BM were identified. Compared to these findings, only 27–29% of CK-positive cells in patients with gastrointestinal carcinomas lacked expression of HLA class I molecules (53), which may explain the predilection of breast cancer for bone metastasis. Consequently, down-regulation of HLA class molecules appears to be an effective mechanism to escape from the anti-tumour immune defence mediated by cytotoxic T lymphocytes. In addition, the overall incidence of HLA negative tumour cells in BM is higher than that reported for the respective primary tumours (83), an observation which further supports the latter assumption that down-regulation of HLA class I molecules may confer a selective survival advantage to CK-positive cells.

3.5 Epithelial Cell Adhesion Molecules

To disseminate in blood and lymphatic vessels tumour cells need coordinated initiation of tumour cell emigration from the primary location to secondary sites. This initial step of metastasis is mediated by flexible adhesive interactions of metastatic cells with different cell types (84). Loss of homotypic adhesion is one of the first actions required for successful disseminating of tumour cells (85).

In epithelial organs, a network of intercellular adhesive junctions is responsible for the tight integration of an individual cell within the tissue (86). The adherens junction complex is organised around the transmembrane E-cadherin protein that organises a complex of cytoplasmatic proteins, including α-catenin, β-catenin and plakoglobin, a β-catenin relative found in desmosomes (86). The cadherin-catenin complex mediates adhesion, cytoskeletal anchoring and signalling. Catenins can also form a complex with the product of the tumour suppressor gene APC, which mediates transmission of a growth regulatory signal (87). To study the expression of plakoglobin on tumour cells, we employed our double marker assay. We found that among the first 25 BM samples admitted to this study, in 17 (68%) samples there was no expression of plakoglobin detectable (Table 3). On the other hand, microaggregates of carcinoma cells present in BM appear to express plakoglobin. Therefore, it is conceivable that down-regulation of plakoglobin expression participates in mechanisms that determine the disseminative capacity of an individual carcinoma cell, whereas the up-regulation of expression might be necessary for solid metastasis formation at the secondary site.

Moreover, another epithelial cell adhesion molecule, EpCAM, also called 17-1A antigen and encoded by the GA-733-2 gene, is found to be present in the great majority of carcinomas and has been employed as a tumour marker (88). Applying our double marker assay, we were able to show a presumably modulated, differential expression of EpCAM on CK-positive cells. Micrometastatic breast cancer cells in BM were found to be EpCAM-positive in 23 (74%) of 31 cases (Table 3). Down-regulation of EpCAM expression might permit tumour cells to escape from contact-mediated controls within the primary tumour, while re-expression at the secondary site might facilitate organ-specific homing of disseminated tumour cells. Consequently, CK-positive cells expressing EpCAM might represent suitable targets for antibody-based therapy.

4. IMPLICATIONS FOR ADJUVANT ANTI-CANCER THERAPY

The efficacy of adjuvant breast cancer therapy can only be assessed retrospectively, employing complex clinical trials following an observation period of at least five years. Therefore, progress in this form of therapy is extremely slow. Moreover, it is very difficult to adapt therapy to the individual need of each patient. Consequently, the importance of a surrogate marker assay that may permit the immediate assessment of therapy-induced cytotoxic effects on residual cancer cells is obvious. Therefore, a follow-up BM aspiration is a feasible option for maintaining MRD during anti-cancer therapy.

New opportunities for specific treatment of cancer residues have been opened by cytotoxic antibodies (89). To maintain the efficacy of this tumour-specific approach, it will be expedient to determine the individual expression pattern of tumour-associated cell-surface targets on disseminated tumour cells

(50), since this pattern may be rather heterogeneous due to the known genetic instability of epithelial cancers. Applying double marker immunoassays combined with the choice of appropriate tumour-specific targets may allow us to establish a surrogate assay for therapeutic efficacy, as demonstrated by the specific elimination of target-positive tumour cells. In a pilot study on 10 breast cancer patients with advanced tumour stages (90), we have been able to show the feasibility of such an approach. Follow-up BM aspirations before and following the administration of a single dose of 500 mg edrecolomab (17-1A antibody) revealed both the reduction of CK-positive and EpCAM-positive/CK-positive tumour cells in all cases examined. To exclude anti-tumour activity other than the one evoked by the applied antibody, we determined the tumour cell number after 5–7 days post treatment, as well as excluded patients with concomitant anti-tumour treatment. Therefore, it is likely that the observed reduction or eradication of CK-positive cells was an effect of the infused antibody.

Schlimok *et al.* presented in another randomised pilot study (91) 40 patients with breast cancer treated with 6×100 mg antibody ABL 364, which is directed to the Lewis Y (Le^Y) blood group precursor carbohydrate antigen (92) versus placebo infusion. CK-positive cells in BM were monitored on days 15 and 60 after initiation of treatment. Even in patients with extremely low number of CK-positive cells (1–11 per 4×10^5 MNC), a tendency for reduction of CK-positive cells was seen after antibody therapy. Significant data, however, were only obtained from the 10 breast cancer patients who displayed an initial cell count of more than 20 CK-positive cells per 4×10^5 MNC. Of the 7 patients treated with antibody, 5 showed a distinct reduction or eradication of CK-positive/Le^Y-positive cells (96–100%), while in 2 patients with CK-positive but Le^Y-negative cells no response was registered. Similarly, in the 3 patients receiving human serum albumin no significant tumour cell reduction was observed. The marked antibody-dependent cellular cytotoxicity and complement-dependent cytotoxicity of the antibody ABL 364 shown in *ex vivo* experiments with serum of treated patients (92) led to the postulation that the observed disappearance of tumour cells from BM was antibody-dependent.

Though these studies may be preliminary, they point to a new approach towards a more rational selection of antibodies for adjuvant studies in minimal residual disease. Recent improvements of the cytokeratin assay (3) allow a more precise quantification of the individual tumour load. Thus, the proposed use of CK-positive cells as surrogate markers for the prediction of therapeutic response may become more effective. Clinical studies are now required to evaluate whether the eradication of CK-positive cells translates into a longer disease-free and overall survival. Availability of such a surrogate marker would considerably enhance our abilities to rationally design new therapies directed towards minimal residual disease.

Current cytotoxic chemotherapy regimes might fail to eliminate dormant, non-proliferating tumour cells, which may explain metastatic relapse even after high-dose chemotherapy. Three studies on breast cancer patients undergoing various regimens of high-dose chemotherapy with autologous stem cell transplantation described the presence of cytokeratin-positive cells in 14 (48%), 15 (83%), and 3 (30%) BM specimens obtained after completion of treatment, with the majority of patients being in complete remission (93–95). Therefore, complementary strategies, such as antibody-based immunotherapy, need to be considered. Hempel *et al.* (95), who treated patients with disseminated CK-positive cells resistant to HD chemotherapy with additional 17-1A antibody (edrecolomab), succeeded in eliminating these cells, and avoidance of early metastatic relapse in 2 of 3 individuals. Interestingly, residual CK-positive cells in both patients yielded co-expression of EpCAM, while the respective cells of the third patient were EpCAM-negative (95).

The successful treatment of metastatic breast cancer with a humanised monoclonal antibody directed against the $p185^{erb\text{-}B2}$-growth factor receptor in combination with chemotherapy has been demonstrated in clinical trials by Baselga *et al.* (10) and Slamon *et al.* (9). These trials are among the first studies in breast cancer patients displaying a biological effect of unconjugated recombinant antibody against established solid tumours. However, the relatively low objective response rates point out that other aspects need to be taken into account. Jain *et al.* previously demonstrated that the relatively high intra-tumour oncotic pressure represents a physiological barrier to deliver monoclonal antibodies and other macromolecules to solid tumours (96). Consequently, a major consideration for the successful application of antibody therapy is the choice of the appropriate disease stage in which the tumour cells are accessible for intravenously administered immunoglobulins (82).

There may be a considerable heterogeneity in the expression pattern of potential immunotherapeutic target antigens determined by the well-known genomic instability of neoplastic cells (89). In addition, in a recent study, we investigated the pattern of tumour-associated antigens, including EpCAM, Le^{Y} and $p185^{erb\text{-}B2}$, expressed on BM micrometastases in breast cancer patients (50). Despite a relatively high incidence of antigen co-expression, our analysis revealed that the number of cells with antigen co-expression per total number of detectable tumour cells varied considerably. These findings indicate a heterogeneous expression pattern of the investigated antigens. To cope with this antigen heterogeneity a combination of antibodies directed to independently expressed antigens should be more efficient than a single agent (50). Since considerable recent progress achieved translation of antibody-based immunological therapies from the laboratory to the clinic, the adjuvant trials initiated have supported the potential of the selective targeting approach for cancer therapy (97). In this context, the possibility to perform follow-up BM aspirations and blood sampling may facilitate the monitoring of the therapeutic efficacy against residual tumour cells.

5. CONCLUSION

The fact that the biological structures and properties of occult micrometastatic cells have so far been barely investigated has been particularly disturbing in patients who remain free of cancer relapse despite the presence of disseminated tumour cells at the time of diagnosis. The presented overview of currently available data indicates that CK-positive micrometastatic tumour cells represent a dormant and selected population of cancer cells, which, however, still express a considerable degree of heterogeneity (8, 50). With the development of new techniques like single-cell PCR (98, 99) and the *in vitro* expansion of micrometastatic cells (100, 101), it will be possible to determine the characteristic genotype features of those cells. Subsequently, large multi-centre trials will be needed to relate biological findings to specified clinical outcomes.

The outlined current strategies for characterisation of cancer micrometastases might help to design and control new therapeutic strategies for secondary prevention of metastatic relapse in patients with operable primary carcinomas. Minimal residual disease offers the advantage of a small burden of dispersed tumour cells which are more accessible to intravenously applied drugs than gross metastases. In view of the dormant nature of micrometastatic cells in BM (8), therapies that are also directed against quiescent cells, such as antibody-based immunotherapy, might be complementary to chemotherapy.

REFERENCES

1. Pantel K, Cote RJ, Fodstad Ø. Detection and clinical importance of micrometastatic disease. J Natl Cancer Inst. 1999;91:1113–24.
2. Schlimok G, Funke I, Holzmann B, Göttlinger HG, Schmidt G, Häuser H *et al.* Micrometastatic cancer cells in bone marrow: in vitro detection with anti-cytokeratin and in vivo labeling with anti-17-1A monoclonal antibodies. Proc Natl Acad Sci USA. 1987;84:8672–6.
3. Pantel K, Schlimok G, Angstwurm M, Weckermann C, Schmaus W, Gath H *et al.* Methodological analysis of immunocytochemical screening for disseminated epithelial tumor cells in bone marrow. J Hematother. 1994;3:165–73.
4. Braun S, Pantel K, Müller P, Janni W, Hepp F, Kentenich CRM *et al.* Cytokeratin-positive cells in the bone marrow and survival of patients with stage I, II or III breast cancer. N Engl J Med. 2000;342:525–33.
5. Mansi JL, Berger U, Easton D, McDonnell T, Redding WH, Gazet JC *et al.* Micrometastases in bone marrow in patients with primary breast cancer: evaluation as an early predictor of bone metastases. Brit Med J. 1987;295:1093–6.
6. Overgaard M, Hansen PS, Overgaard J, Rose C, Andersson M, Bach F *et al.* Postoperative radiotherapy in high-risk premenopausal women with breast cancer who receive adjuvant chemotherapy. N Engl J Med. 1997;337:949–55.
7. Braun S, Pantel K. Prognostic significance of micrometastatic bone marrow involvement. Breast Cancer Res Treat. 1998;52:201–16.
8. Pantel K, Schlimok G, Braun S, Kutter D, Schaller G, Funke I *et al.* Differential expression of proliferation-associated molecules in individual micrometastatic carcinoma cells. J Natl Cancer Inst. 1993;85:1419–24.
9. Slamon JD, Leyland-Jones B, Shak S, Paton V, Bajamonde A, Fleming T *et al.* Use of chemotherapy plus a monoclonal antibody against HER2 for metastatic breast cancer that overexpresses HER2. N Engl J Med. 2001;344:783–92.

10. Baselga J, Tripathy D, Mendelsohn J, Baughman, Benz CC, Dantis L *et al.* Phase II study of weekly intravenous recombinant humanized anti-p185Her2 monoclonal antibody in patients with Her2/neu-overexpressing metastatic breast cancer. J Clin Oncol. 1996;14:737–44.
11. Braun S, Rosenberg R, Thorban S, Harbeck N. Implications of occult metastatic cells for systemic cancer treatment in patients with breast or gastrointestinal cancer. Semin Surg Oncol. 2001;20:334–46.
12. Schwarz G. Cytomorphology and cell yield in a new cytocentrifugal technique allowing the collection of the cell-free supernatant. Lab Med. 1991;15:45–50.
13. Dearnaley D, Ormerod M, Sloane J. Micrometastases in breast cancer: long-term follow-up of the first patient cohort. Eur J Cancer. 1991;27:236–9.
14. Dearnaley D, Sloane J, Ormerod M, Steele K, Coombes R, Clink H *et al.* Increased detection of mammary carcinoma cells in marrow smears using antisera to epithelial membrane antigen. Brit J Cancer. 1983;44:85–90.
15. Redding WH, Coombes RC, Monagham P, Clink HMD, Imrie SF, Dearnaley DP *et al.* Detection of micrometastases in patients with primary breast cancer. Lancet. 1983;2:1271–4.
16. Funke I, Schraut W. Meta-analysis of studies on bone marrow micrometastases: an independent prognostic impact remains to be substantiated. J Clin Oncol. 1998; 16:557–66.
17. Gebauer G, Fehm T, Merkle E, Beck EP, Lang N, Jager W. Epithelial cells in bone marrow of breast cancer patients at time of primary surgery: clinical outcome during long-term follow-up. J Clin Oncol. 2001;19:3669–74.
18. Braun S, Cevatli BS, Assemi C, Janni W, Kentenich CRM, Schindlbeck C *et al.* Comparative analysis of micrometastasis to the bone marrow and lymph nodes of node-negative breast cancer patients receiving no adjuvant therapy. J Clin Oncol. 2001;19:1468–75.
19. Gerber B, Krause A, Muller H, Richter D, Reimer T, Makovitzky J *et al.* Simultaneous immunohistochemical detection of tumor cells in lymph nodes and bone marrow aspirates in breast cancer and its correlation with other prognostic factors. J Clin Oncol. 2001;19:960–71.
20. Mansi JL, Gogas H, Bliss JM, Gazet JC, Berger U, Coombes RC. Outcome of primary-breast-cancer patients with micrometastases: a long-term follow-up. Lancet. 1999;354:197–202.
21. Landys K, Persson S, Kovarik J, Hultborn R, Holmberg E. Prognostic value of bone marrow biopsy in operable breast cancer patients at the time of initial diagnosis: results of a 20-year median follow-up. Breast Cancer Res Treat. 1998; 49:27–33.
22. Diel IJ, Kaufmann M, Costa SD, Holle R, von Minckwitz G, Solomayer EF *et al.* Micrometastatic breast cancer cells in bone marrow at primary surgery: prognostic value in comparison with nodal status. J Natl Cancer Inst. 1996;88:1652–64.
23. Harbeck N, Untch M, Pache L, Eiermann W. Tumour cell detection in the bone marrow of breast cancer patients at primary therapy: results of a 3-year median follow-up. Brit J Cancer. 1994;69:566–71.
24. Cote RJ, Rosen PP, Lesser ML, Old LJ, Osborne MP. Prediction of early relapse in patients with operable breast cancer by detection of occult bone marrow micrometastases. J Clin Oncol. 1991;9:1749–56.
25. Untch M, Kahlert S, Funke I, Boettcher B, Konecny G, Nestle-Kraemling C *et al.* Detection of cytokeratin 18-positive cells in bone marrow of breast cancer patients: no prediction of bad outcome. Proc Amer Soc Clin Oncol. 1999;18:639a (abstr #2472).

26. Molino A, Pelosi G, Turazza M, Sperotto L, Bonetti A, Nortilli R *et al.* Bone marrow micrometastases in 109 breast cancer patients: correlations with clinical and pathological features. Breast Cancer Res Treat. 1997;42:23–30.
27. Funke I, Fries S, Rolle M, Heiss MM, Untch M, Bohmert H *et al.* Comparative analyses of bone marrow micrometastases in breast and gastric cancer. Int J Cancer. 1996;65:755–61.
28. Courtemanche DJ, Worth AJ, Coupland RW, Rowell JL, MacFarlane JK. Monoclonal antibody LICR-LON-M8 does not predict the outcome of operable breast cancer. Can J Surg. 1991;34:21–6.
29. Singletary SE, Larry L, Trucker SL, Spitzer G. Detection of micrometastatic tumor cells in bone marrow of breast carcinoma patients. J Surg Oncol. 1991;47:32–6.
30. Mathieu MC, Friedman S, Bosq J, Caillou B, Spielmann M, Travagli JP *et al.* Immunohistochemical staining of bone marrow biopsies for detection of occult metastasis in breast cancer. Breast Cancer Res Treat. 1990;15:21–6.
31. Salvadori B, Squicciarini P, Rovini D, Orefice S, Andreola S, Rilke F *et al.* Use of monoclonal antibody MBr1 to detect micrometastases in bone marrow specimens of breast cancer patients. Eur J Cancer. 1990;26:865–7.
32. Porro G, Menard S, Tagliabue E, Orefice S, Salvadori B, Squicciarini P *et al.* Monoclonal antibody detection of carcinoma cells in bone marrow biopsy specimens from breast cancer patients. Cancer. 1988;61:2407–11.
33. Braun S, Müller M, Hepp F, Schlimok G, Riethmüller G, Pantel K. Re: Micrometastatic breast cancer cells in bone marrow at primary surgery: prognostic value in comparison with nodal status. J Natl Cancer Inst. 1998;90:1099–100.
34. Datta YH, Adams PT, Drobyski WR. Sensitive detection of occult breast cancer by the reverse-transcriptase polymerase chain reaction. J Clin Oncol. 1994;12:475–82.
35. Fields KK, Elfenbein GJ, Trudeau WL, Perlinss JB, Jansen WE, Moscinski LC. Clinical significance of bone marrow metastases as detected using polymerase chain reaction in patients with breast cancer undergoing high-dose chemotherapy and autologous bone marrow transplantation. J Clin Oncol. 1996;14:1868–76.
36. Vannucchi AM, Bosi A, Glinz S, Pacini P, Linari S, Saccardi R *et al.* Evaluation of breast tumour cell contamination in the bone marrow and leukapheresis collections by RT-PCR for cytokeratin-19 mRNA. Brit J Haematol. 1998;103(3):610–7.
37. Slade MJ, Smith BM, Sinnett HD, Cross NCP, Coombes RC. Quantitative polymerase chain reaction for the detection of micrometastases in patients with breast cancer. J Clin Oncol. 1999;17:870–9.
38. Mapara MY, Körner IJ, Hildebrandt M, Bargou R, Krahl D, Reichardt P *et al.* Monitoring of tumor cell purging after highly efficient immunomagnetic selection of CD34 cells from leukapheresis products in breast cancer patients: comparison of immunocytochemical tumor cell staining and reverse transcriptase-polymerase chain reaction. Blood. 1997;89:337–44.
39. Zach O, Kasparu H, Krieger O, Hehenwarter W, Girschikofsky M, Lutz D. Detection of circulating mammary carcinoma cells in the peripheral blood of breast cancer patients via a nested reverse transcriptase polymerase chain reaction assay for mammaglobin mRNA. J Clin Oncol. 1999;17:2015–19.
40. Bettelheim R, Price KN, Gelber RD, Davis BW, Castiglione M, Neville AM. Prognostic importance of occult axillary lymph node micrometastases from breast cancers. Lancet. 1990;335:1565–8.
41. De Mascarel I, Bonichon F, Coindre JM, Trojani M. Prognostic significance of breast cancer axillary lymph node micrometastases assessed by two special techniques: reevaluation with longer follow up. Brit J Cancer. 1992;66:523–7.

42. Bussolati G, Gugliotta P, Morra I, Pietribiasi F, Berardengo E. The immunohistochemical detection of lymph node metastases from infiltrating lobular carcinoma. Br J Cancer. 1986;54:631–6.
43. Nasser IA, Lee AKC, Bosari S, Saganich R, Heatley G, Silverman ML. Occult axillary lymph node metastases in 'node-negative' breast carcinoma. Hum Pathol. 1993;24:950–7.
44. McGuckin MA, Cummings MC, Walsh MD, Hohn BG, Bennett IC, Wright RG. Occult axillary node metastases in breast cancer: their detection and prognostic significance. Br J Cancer. 1996;73:88–95.
45. Cote RJ, Peterson HF, Chaiwun B, Gelber RD, Goldhirsch A, Castiglione-Gertsch M *et al.* Role of immunohistochemical detection of lymph-node metastases in management of breast cancer. Lancet. 1999;354:896–900.
46. Noguchi S, Aihara T, Nakamori S, Motomura K, Inaji H, Imaoka S *et al.* The detection of breast cancer micrometastases in axillary lymph nodes by means of reverse transcriptase-polymerase chain reaction. Cancer. 1994;74:1595–600.
47. Schönfeld A, Luqmani Y, Sinnett HD, Shousha S, Coombes RC. Keratin 19 mRNA measurement to detect micrometastases in lymph nodes in breast cancer patients. Brit J Cancer. 1996;74:1639–42.
48. Ridell B, Landys K. Incidence and histopathology of metastases of mammary carcinoma in biopsies from the posterior iliac creast. Cancer. 1979;44:1782–8.
49. Fisher B, Fisher ER, Guzman C, Copeland CE, Caceres E. The dissemination of subcutaneously inoculated tumor cell suspensions. Arch Surg. 1968;98:347–51.
50. Braun S, Hepp F, Sommer HL, Pantel K. Tumor antigen heterogeneity of disseminated breast cancer cells: implications for immunotherapy of minimal residual disease. Int J Cancer (Pred Oncol). 1999;84:1–5.
51. Pantel K, Aignherr C, Köllermann J, Caprano J, Riethmüller G, Köllermann MW. Immunocytochemical detection of isolated tumor cells in bone marrow of patients with untreated stage C prostatic cancer. Eur J Cancer. 1995;31A: 1627–32.
52. Riesenberg R, Oberneder R, Kriegmair M, Epp M, Bitzer U, Hofstetter A *et al.* Immunocytochemical double staining of cytokeratin and prostate specific antigen in individual prostatic tumor cells. Histochem. 1993;99:61–6.
53. Pantel K, Schlimok G, Kutter D, Schaller G, Genz T, Wiebecke B *et al.* Frequent down-regulation of major histocompatibility class I antigen expression on individual micrometastatic carcinoma cells. Cancer Res. 1991;51:4712–15.
54. Fox SB, Leek RD, Bliss J, Mansi JL, Gusterson B, Gatter KC *et al.* Association of tumor angiogenesis with bone marrow micrometastases in breast cancer. J Natl Cancer Inst. 1997;89:1044–9.
55. Maehara Y, Hasuda S, Abe T, Oki E, Kakeji Y, Ohno S *et al.* Tumor angiogenesis and micrometastasis in bone marrow of patients with early gastric cancer. Clin Cancer Res. 1998;4:2129–34.
56. McCulloch P, Choy A, Martin L. Association between tumour angiogenesis and tumour cell shedding into effluent venous blood during breast cancer surgery. Lancet. 1995;346:1334–5.
57. Choy A, McCulloch P. Induction of tumor cell shedding into effluent venous blood during breast cancer surgery. Brit J Cancer. 1996;73:79–82.
58. Ménard S, Squicciarini P, Luini A, Sacchini V, Rovini D, Tagliabue E *et al.* Immunodetection of bone marrow micrometastases in breast carcinoma patients and its correlation with tumor prognostic features. Brit J Cancer. 1994;69: 1126–9.

59. Martignone S, Ménard S, Bufalino R, Cascinelli N, Pellegrini R, Tagliabue E *et al.* Prognostic significance of the 67-kilodalton laminin receptor expression in human breast carcinomas. J Natl Cancer Inst. 1993;85:398–402.
60. Gerdes J, Lemke H, Baisch H, Wacker HH, Schwab U, Stein H. Cell cycle analysis of a cell proliferation-associated human nuclear antigen defined by the monoclonal antibody *Ki-67*. J Immunol. 1984;133(4):1710–15.
61. Freeman JW, Busch RK, Gyorkey F, Gyorkey P, Ross BE, Busch H. Identification and characterization of a human proliferation-associated nucleolar antigen with a molecular weight of 120,000 expressed in early G1 phase. Cancer Res. 1988;48:1244–51.
62. Fidler IJ, Radinsky R. Genetic control of cancer metastasis. J Natl Cancer Inst. 1990;82:166–8.
63. Liotta LA, Steeg PS, Stetler-Stevenson WG. Cancer metastasis and angiogenesis: an imbalance of positive and negative regulation. Cell. 1991;64:327–36.
64. Price JE, Aukerman SL, Ananthaswamy N, McIntyre BW, Schackert G, Fidler IJ. Metastatic potential of cloned murine melanoma cells transfected with activated c-Ha-ras. Cancer Res. 1989;49:4274–81.
65. Pantel K, Schmaus W, Schlimok G, Riethmüller G. p53 immunostaining of megakaryocytes is preferentially observed in patients with epithelial malignancies. Blood. 1993;82:610a (abstract).
66. Schlimok G, Riethmüller G. Detection, characterization and tumorigenicity of tumor cells in human bone marrow. Semin Cancer Biol. 1990;1:207–15.
67. Allgayer H, Heiss MM, Riesenberg R, Gruetzner KU, Tarabichi A, Babic R *et al.* Urokinase plasminogen activator receptor (uPA-R): one potential characteristic of metastatic phenotypes in minimal residual tumor disease. Cancer Res. 1997;57:1394–9.
68. Iggo R, Gatter K, Bartek J, Lane D, Harris AL. Increased expression of mutant forms of *p53* oncogene in primary lung cancer. Lancet. 1990;335:675–9.
69. Hall PA, Ray A, Lemoine NR, Midley CA, Krausz T, Lane DP. p53 immunostaining as a marker of malignant disease in diagnostic cytopathology. Lancet. 1991;338:531.
70. Slamon JD, Godolphin W, Jones LA, Holt JA, Wong SG, Keith DE *et al.* Studies of the HER-2/neu proto-oncogene in human breast cancer and ovarian cancer. Science. 1989;244:707–12.
71. Bianchi S, Paglierani M, Zampi G, Cardona G, Cataliotti L, Bonardi R *et al.* Prognostic significance of c-erbB-2 expression in node negative breast cancer. Brit J Cancer. 1993;67(3):625–9.
72. Berger MS, Locher GW, Saurer S, Gullick WJ, Waterfield MD, Groner B *et al.* Correlation of c-erbB-2 gene amplification and protein expression in human breast carcinoma with nodal status and nuclear grading. Cancer Res. 1988;48(5):1238–43.
73. Tiwari RK, Borgen PI, Wong GY, Cordon CC, Osborne MP. HER-2/neu amplification and overexpression in primary human breast cancer is associated with early metastasis. Anticancer Res. 1992;12:419–25.
74. Varley JM, Swallow JE, Brammar WJ, Whittaker JL, Walker RA. Alterations to either c-erbB-2(neu) or c-myc proto-oncogenes in breast carcinomas correlate with poor short-term prognosis. Oncogene. 1987;1:423–30.
75. Venter DJ, Tuzi NL, Kumar S, Gullick WJ. Overexpression of the *c-erb-B-2* oncoprotein in human breast carcinomas: immunhistochemical assessment correlates with gene amplification. Lancet. 1987;2:69–72.
76. Braun S, Heumos I, Schlimok G, Schaller G, Riethdorf L, Riethmüller G *et al.* ErbB2 over-expression on occult metastatic cells in bone marrow predicts poor clinical outcome of stage I-III breast cancer patients. Cancer Res. 2001;61:1890–5.

77. Taylor-Papadimitriou J. Oncogene signalling epithelial polarity and metastatic phenotype. In: The Lancet Conference, 1994; Brugge, Belgium; 1994, p. 7.
78. Hoffman M. New clue found to oncogene's role in breast cancer. Science. 1992; 256:1129.
79. Lupu R, Colomer R, Kannan B, Lippman ME. Characterization of a growth factor that binds exclusively to the erbB2 receptor and induces cellular responses. Proc Natl Acad Sci USA. 1992;89:2287–91.
80. Peles E, Bacus SS, Koski RA, Lu HS, Wen D, Ogden SG *et al.* Isolation of the neu/HER-2 stimulatory ligand: a 44 kD glycoprotein that induces differentiation of mammary tumor cells. Cell. 1992;69:205–16.
81. Brandt B, Roetger A, Heidl S, Jackisch C, Lelle RJ, Assmann G *et al.* Isolation of blood-borne epithelium derived c-erb-B2 oncoprotein-positive clustered cells from peripheral blood of breast cancer patients. Int J Cancer. 1998;76:824–8.
82. Riethmüller G, Johnson JP. Monoclonal antibodies in the detection and therapy of micrometastatic epithelial cancer. Curr Opin Immunol. 1992;4:647–55.
83. Hämmerling G, Maschek V, Sturmhöfel K, Momburg F. Regulation and functional role of MHC expression on tumors. In: Melchers F, editor. Prog. Immunol. Berlin: Springer; 1989, p. 1071–8.
84. Behrens J, Frixen U, Schipper J, Weidner M, Birchmeier W. Cell adhesion in invasion and metastasis. Semin Cell Biol. 1992;3:169–78.
85. Hart IR, Goode NT, Wilson RE. Molecular aspects of the metastatic cascade. Biochem Biophys Acta. 1989;989:65–84.
86. Schwarz MA, Owaribe K, Kartenbeck J, Franke WW. Desmosomes and hemidesmosomes: constitutive molecular components. Annu Rev Cell Biol. 1990;6:461–91.
87. Pfeifer M. Cancer, catenins, and cuticle pattern: a complex connection. Science. 1993;262:667.
88. Göttlinger HG, Funke I, Johnson JP, Gokel JM, Riethmüller G. The epithelial cell surface antigen 17-1A, a target for antibody-mediated tumor therapy: its biochemical nature, tissue distribution and recognition by different monoclonal antibodies. Int J Cancer. 1986;38:47–53.
89. Dillman RO. Antibodies as cytotoxic therapy. J Clin Oncol. 1994;12:1497–515.
90. Braun S, Hepp F, Kentenich CRM, Janni W, Pantel K, Riethmüller G *et al.* Monoclonal antibody therapy with edrecolomab in breast cancer patients: monitoring of elimination of disseminated cytokeratin-positive tumor cells in bone marrow. Clin Cancer Res. 1999;5:3999–4004.
91. Schlimok G, Pantel K, Loibner H, Fackler-Schwalbe I, Riethmüller G. Reduction of metastatic carcinoma cells in bone marrow by intravenously administered monoclonal antibody: towards a novel surrogate test to monitor adjuvant therapies of solid tumours. Eur J Cancer. 1995;31A:1799–803.
92. Scholz D, Lubeck M, Loibner H. Biological activity in the human system of isotype variants of oligosaccharide Y-specific murine monoclonal antibodies. Cancer Immunol Immunother. 1991;33:153–7.
93. Kruger WH, Kroger N, Togel F, Renges H, Badbaran A, Hornung R *et al.* Disseminated breast cancer cells prior to and after high-dose therapy. J Hematother Stem Cell Res. 2001;10:681–9.
94. Hohaus S, Funk L, Martin S, Schlenk R, Abdallah A, Hahn U *et al.* Stage III and oestrogen receptor negativity are associated with poor prognosis after adjuvant high-dose therapy in high-risk breast cancer. Br J Cancer. 1999;79:1500–7.

95. Hempel D, Müller P, Oruzio D, Ehnle S, Schlimok G. Adoptive immunotherapy with monoclonal antibody 17-1A to reduce minimal residual disease in breast cancer patients after high-dose chemotherapy. Blood. 1997;90 Suppl. 1:379B, abstract #4454.
96. Jain RK. Physiological barriers to delivery of monoclonal antibodies and other macromolecules in tumors. Cancer Res. 1990;50:2741–51.
97. Scott AM, Welt S. Antibody-based immunological therapies. Curr Opin Immunol. 1997;9:717–22.
98. Klein CA, Schmidt-Kittler O, Schardt JA, Pantel K, Speicher MR, Riethmüller G. Comparative genomic hybridization, loss of heterozygosity, and DNA sequence analysis of single cells. Proc Natl Acad Sci USA. 1999;96:4494–99.
99. Klein CA, Seidl S, Petat-Dutter K, Offner S, Geigl JB, Schmidt-Kittler O *et al.* Combined transcriptome and genome analysis of singel micrometastatic cells. Nat Biotech. 2002;20:387–92.
100. Putz E, Witter K, Offner S, Stosiek P, Zippelius A, Johnson JP *et al.* Phenotypic characteristics of cell lines derived from disseminated cancer cells in bone marrow of patients with solid epithelial tumors: establishment of working models for human micrometastases. Cancer Res. 1999;59:241–8.
101. Pantel K, Dickmanns A, Zippelius A, Klein C, Shi J, Hoechtlen-Vollmar W *et al.* Establishment of micrometastatic carcinoma cell lines: a novel source of tumor cell vaccines. J Natl Cancer Inst. 1995;87:1162–8.

Chapter 4

PROGNOSIS OF MINIMAL RESIDUAL DISEASE IN BONE MARROW, BLOOD AND LYMPH NODES IN BREAST CANCER

Debra Hawes[1], A. Munro Neville[2], Richard J. Cote[1]

[1]*Keck School of Medicine at the University of Southern California/Kenneth Norris Comprehensive Cancer Center, Los Angeles, California, USA;* [2]*Ludwig Institute for Cancer Research, London, UK*

Abstract
The most important factor affecting the outcome of patients with invasive cancers is whether the tumor has spread, either regionally (to regional lymph nodes) or systemically (to the bone marrow). However, a proportion of patients with no evidence of systemic dissemination will develop recurrent disease after primary therapy. Clearly, these patients had occult systemic spread of disease that was undetectable by methods routinely employed (careful pathological, clinical, biochemical and radiological evaluation). This early dissemination of tumor cells is known as occult metastases (or micrometastases). In addition, the success of adjuvant therapy is assumed to stem from its ability to eradicate occult metastases before they become clinically evident. Therefore, methods for the detection of occult metastases in patients with the earliest stage of cancer, i.e., prior to detection of metastases by any other clinical or pathological analysis, have received a great deal of attention. This chapter focuses on the detection and significance of occult metastatic cells in the peripheral blood bone marrow and lymph nodes of patients with breast cancer.

1. OCCULT METASTASIS

The goal of diagnostic surgical pathology is twofold: to arrive at the specific diagnosis (benign or malignant and cell of origin) and to stage the tumor (1). These are the two important parameters that determine the rational treatment of any type of tumor. Using pathological criteria in conjunction with clinical parameters, the pathologist and the clinician attempt to determine the outcome of a patient. Staging criteria are used to evaluate almost any type of solid tumor and are important not only in predicting prognosis, but also in selecting appropriate therapy.

The majority of patients with newly diagnosed breast cancer have operable disease, and these patients are considered potentially curable. However, 35% to 40% of these patients, including up to 24% of patients with no evidence of metastasis at the time of diagnosis, develop recurrent disease after primary

K. Pantel (ed.), Micrometastasis, 67–85.

therapy. The most reliable prognostic parameters (lymph node status and tumor size) cannot predict which particular individual will progress. As a result, several groups have recommended adjuvant treatment for patients with lymph node negative disease. While this is controversial (since the majority of node negative patients will be clinically cured without adjuvant therapy), it is in this group of patients who have minimal occult metastases that adjuvant therapy should be most successful. It would be of great value, therefore, to be able to further discriminate and identify those patients with early-stage disease who are most likely to recur. Detection of occult metastatic cells in these patients could be extremely beneficial in determining prognosis and in making treatment decisions.

1.1 Methods Used for the Detection of Occult Metastases

Several techniques have been used to identify occult metastases. The most important of these include: immunohistochemistry (IHC), flow cytometry, and molecular methods, usually the reverse-transcriptase polymerase chain reaction (RT-PCR) technique. These different methodologies vary in their ability to identify occult metastases, and as well as in their ability to predict outcome. The pros and cons of these techniques are discussed below.

1.1.1 Immunohistochemistry

Following pioneering studies at the Ludwig Institute and Royal Marsden Hospital in London, England (2), a number of groups have used immunohistochemical procedures to identify occult metastatic cancer cells in the peripheral blood bone marrow of patients with cancer. While many of the initial studies focused on breast cancer (2–6), tumors from other organs, such as colon (7–9), prostate (10–13) and lung (14–18), have also been investigated. Immunohistochemical methods are based on the ability of monoclonal antibodies to distinguish between cells of different histogenesis (i.e., epithelial cancer cells vs. hematopoietic cells, and cells of the peripheral blood, bone marrow and lymph nodes (Figures 1 and 2)). The results indicate that it is possible to identify occult metastatic cancer cells in these compartments prior to their detection by routine histologic analyses, and that the presence of these cells may be an important risk factor for disease recurrence.

The most widely used monoclonal antibodies to detect occult metastatic cells are antibodies to epithelial-specific antigens. These antibodies do not react with hematopoietic cells normally present in the peripheral blood, bone marrow and lymph nodes. None of the antibodies used in any study is specific for cancer; all react with normal and malignant epithelial cells. They are useful because they can identify an extrinsic population of epithelial cells in the blood and bone marrow, where there are normally no epithelial elements. The reported sensitivity of the immunohistochemical method ranges from the detection of one epithelial cell in 10,000 (3) to that of two to five epithelial cells in a million hematopoietic cells (3, 6).

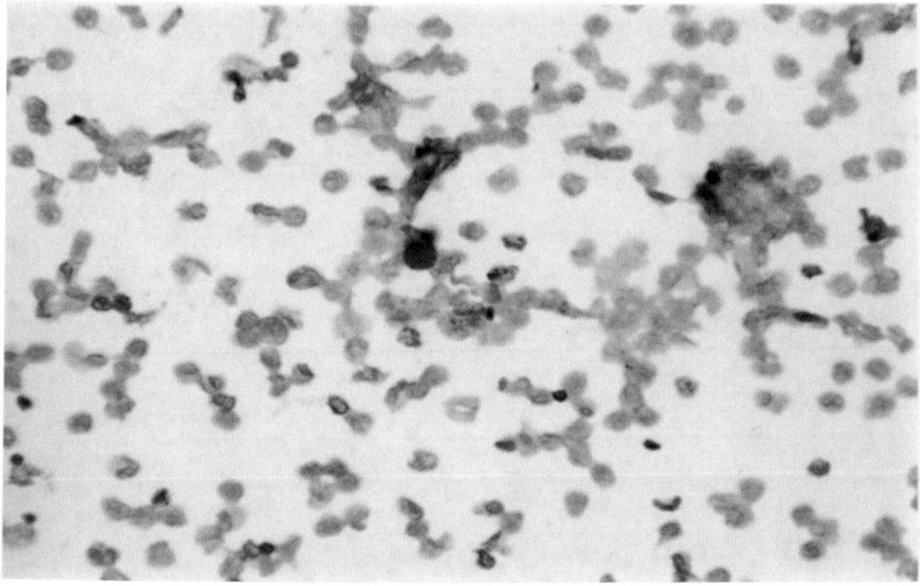

Figure 1. Bone marrow from patient with breast cancer showing a cytokeratin positive tumor cell detected by immunohistochemistry.

1.1.2 Molecular Methods

While immunohistochemical methods are effective in identifying occult metastases in the peripheral blood, bone marrow and lymph nodes of patients with operable breast cancer, these methods are laborious and require considerable technical expertise to perform and interpret. Efforts are under way to develop molecular techniques for the detection of occult metastases. The method usually employed is RT-PCR, which differentiates gene expression between epithelial and lymphoid cells to identify epithelial cancer cells. RT-PCR entails the isolation and reverse transcription of epithelial-specific messenger RNA to complementary-DNA (cDNA), and thereafter, involves PCR-based amplification of the cDNA template between specific primers. This results in a several thousand-fold amplification of the signal, and makes the method theoretically extremely sensitive. These methods are theoretically more sensitive than immunohistochemistry and provide the possibility of automation. Keratin 18 or 19 mRNA that is expressed in epithelial cells has been the most frequent target for amplification to detect occult metastases. Datta *et al.* (1994) (19) used the keratin 19 transcript to identify cancer cells in the bone marrow and peripheral blood of breast cancer patients. It is known that a pseudogene for keratin 19 exists that shares a very high homology with the mature mRNA from the keratin 19 gene. Contamination of DNA in the RNA sample used for reverse transcription can result in amplification of the pseudogene, giving rise to specific 'background' bands in the

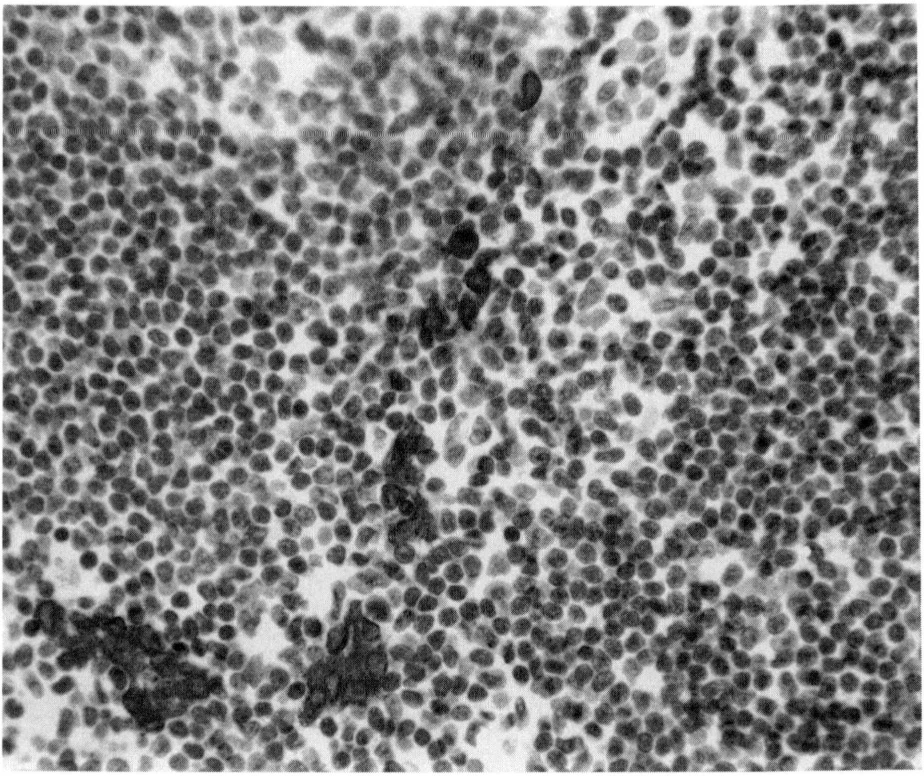

Figure 2. Sentinel lymph node from patient with breast cancer showing cytokeratin positive tumor cells detected by immunohistochemistry that were not detected by routine H&E.

negative controls (known negative bone marrow and blood) (13). Furthermore, the non-epithelial cells may have a low level of expression of epithelial transcripts, leading to background bands. To circumvent this problem, we have attempted to amplify transcripts from epithelial and breast cell-specific genes including carcinoembryonic antigen (CEA), cytokeratin 19 (CK-19), cytokeratin-20 (CK-20), mucin-1 (MUC-1) and gastrointestinal tumor-associated antigen 733.2 (GA733.2), from the blood of healthy donors and lymph nodes from patients without cancer by RT-PCR. CK-20 was the only marker not detected in the lymph nodes or blood from patients without cancer (20).

In addition, Zippelius *et al.* (21) studied the specificity of RT-PCR assays with primers specific for various tumor-associated and organ-specific mRNA species, including prostate-specific antigen (PSA), epithelial glycoprotein-40 (EGP-40) desmoplakin I (DPI I) carcinoembryonic antigen (CEA), *erb*-B2, *erb*-B3 prostate-specific membrane antigen (PSM) and CK18. They looked at the bone marrow from 53 subjects with no epithelial malignancy, as well as bone marrow samples from 53 patients with prostate cancer and 10 patients with breast cancer. They found that seven of the eight markers tested could be detected in a considerable number of bone marrow samples from control patients. In their hands, only PSA mRNA was not detected in any of the 53 control bone marrow samples (21). The known relative non-specificity of these epithelial cell markers has prompted the search for even more specific breast cancer markers. One such candidate currently under investigation is mammoglobin. Mammoglobin, a glycoprotein expressed in the mammary glands of women, as well as in breast cancer cell lines, has been investigated as a potential marker to detect early metastatic breast cancer in the peripheral blood (22–24) of patients with breast cancer. Grunewald *et al.* (22) have examined peripheral blood samples from 12 patients with ductal carcinoma *in situ*, 133 patients with invasive breast cancer, 20 patients with hematological malignancies, 31 healthy volunteers along with tumor samples from 40 patients with invasive breast cancer. Each sample was screened by RT-PCR for mammoglobin (hMAM), epidermal growth factor receptor (EGF-R) and cytokeratin 19 (CK-19). They found that of the blood samples from patients with invasive breast cancer ($n = 133$), 11 (8%) were positive for mammoglobin, while 13 (10%) were positive for EGR-R and 64 (48%) were CK-19 positive. None of the blood samples from patients without cancer was positive for mammoglobin mRNA (22). In summary, the drawbacks of molecular methods include the chance of low level of epithelial gene expression from lymphoid cells that could result in high background, as well as the inability to employ morphologic criteria to confirm the presence of metastatic cells; this has been the case in our studies. However, RT-PCR has been successfully used for the detection of occult metastases to the bone marrow in melanoma and carcinoma of the prostate and colon.

1.1.3 Flow Cytometry

A flow cytometric assay has recently been developed to detect rare cancer cells in the blood and bone marrow (25). The method is reported to be extremely sensitive, with an ability to detect one positive cell in ten million blood cells in a model system; this is in contrast to all other reports on the sensitivity of flow cytometry (26). One major disadvantage of most flow cytometric systems is the inability to morphologically characterize the cells constituting the 'positive' events. However, by employing sophisticated cell-sorting technologies, in which the extrinsic cell population can be captured for subsequent morphologic evaluation, the specificity of tumor cell detection might be improved.

With this overview, the following sections will describe the significance of detecting occult metastatic cells in the peripheral blood, bone marrow and lymph nodes from patients with breast cancer.

2. PERIPHERAL BLOOD VERSUS BONE MARROW

Peripheral blood would clearly be the most convenient sample site for studies to detect occult metastatic cells. Unfortunately, the yield of occult metastatic cells from peripheral blood is extremely low. Redding *et al.* (2) found that 28.2% of patients with breast cancer showed extrinsic cancer cells in their bone marrow, but only 2.7% of these patients had detectable cells in their peripheral blood. It is not clear why tumor cells are detected less commonly in peripheral blood than in bone marrow. The bone marrow vasculature consists of a unique sinusoidal system that may simply act as a filter that traps or concentrates malignant cells. The marrow environment may provide a more favorable support system for tumor cell proliferation than does blood. One may also speculate that cancer cells that are released into the systemic circulation represent a small sub-population of cells with altered expression of cell adhesion molecules. Whatever the reason, bone marrow appears to offer the maximum opportunity to detect cancer cells that have been released into the blood. Therefore, the majority of studies to detect occult metastatic cells in the systemic circulation have investigated bone marrow as a site of spread.

2.1 Detection of Occult Metastases in the Peripheral Blood

Assessment of the peripheral blood for the presence of occult metastases has the obvious advantage of being less invasive and easier to obtain than is a bone marrow sample that requires a more invasive procedure to obtain. The major disadvantage, as discussed above, is that it is maybe a less sensitive compartment than bone marrow for the determination of early tumor cell dissemination. For this reason, most of the studies examining the presence of early metastases in the blood have focused on using molecular methods.

Kim *et al.* (27) have examined the peripheral blood samples from 21 patients with primary operable breast cancer, 29 patients with metastatic breast cancer and 21 healthy women by immunohistochemistry following immunomagnetic separation. Tumor cells were not detected in either the healthy women or the women with operable breast cancer. Conversely, 8 of the 29 (28%) women with metastatic breast cancer did have tumor cells in their peripheral blood (27). Slade *et al.* (28) looked at both peripheral blood and bone marrow samples from women with primary breast cancer using RT-PCR for CK-19. They examined 45 peripheral blood and 30 bone marrow samples from patients with non-neoplastic conditions, as well as the peripheral blood and bone marrow samples from 23 patients with primary breast cancer and peripheral blood samples only from 37 patients with metastatic breast cancer. In addition, RT-PCR results were compared to CK-19 positive cells detected by immunohistochemistry. The normal subjects were used to establish cut-off points to determine relative positivity of CK-19. By their criteria, only 3 of 23 (13%) primary breast cancer peripheral blood and none of the control samples were positive. Only 2 of 23 (9%) patients with primary breast cancer showed immunohistochemically detectable cells in the blood; 10 of 23 (43%) showed immunohistochemically detectable cells in the bone marrow. Of 36 patients with metastatic breast cancer, 8 (22%) showed positive results (28).

The prognostic significance of the presence of occult metastatic cells in the peripheral blood with patients with primary carcinoma of the breast, unlike occult metastases in the bone marrow, is uncertain and requires further clinical evaluation and follow-up studies.

2.2 Detection of Occult Metastases in the Bone Marrow in Patients with Breast Cancer

Bone marrow is the single most common site of breast cancer metastasis, and up to 80% of patients with recurrent tumors will develop metastatic lesions in the bone marrow at some point during evolution of their diseases (29); it is also the most frequent initial site of clinically detectable breast cancer metastasis (30). Tumor cells are estimated to be present in the bone marrow of 20% to 45% of patients with primary operable breast cancer (2, 6, 31–34), and 20% to 70% of patients with metastatic breast cancer (35). As with most cancers, the most widely used method to detect occult metastatic cells is immunohistochemistry.

2.2.1 Rate of Detection of Bone Marrow Occult Metastases in Patients with Early Stage Breast Cancer

Because immunohistochemistry is the most widely used (and currently, the most reliable) method for the detection of occult metastases in the bone marrow in breast cancer patients, we have summarized the results from several groups performing immunohistochemical assays using monoclonal antibodies.

The percentage of patients with early-stage breast cancer in whom extrinsic cells were detected in the bone marrow ranges from 16% to 38%. The possible reasons for some of the variations observed include: (i) use of single antibodies to detect extrinsic cells in some of the studies, (ii) differences in patient populations, although all the results were from patients with early-stage disease, (iii) differences in the antibody reactivity with breast cancer cells, and (iv) the presence of antigenic heterogeneity. However, what is evident and striking is that occult metastases in the bone marrow were detected in all of the studies. Furthermore, it is becoming apparent that the rate of detection of occult metastases in the bone marrow in patients with operable breast cancer is approximately 20% to 30% when appropriate antibodies are used. Finally, bone marrow occult metastases can be detected in a proportion of patients with no evidence of metastatic spread.

2.2.2 Detection of Occult Metastases in the Bone Marrow in Patients with Early-Stage Breast Cancer: Clinical Significance

Bone marrow occult metastases have been correlated with known predictors of prognosis in several studies. In our studies (6), extrinsic cells were detected in 27% of node negative patients, and in 41% of node positive patients. On an average, the lymph node negative group had fewer extrinsic cells than the lymph node positive group, suggesting a trend towards a greater metastatic tumor burden in patients with lymph node metastases.

The presence of occult metastases in the bone marrow has been correlated with pathologic tumor, node, metastasis (TNM) stage in breast cancer. In our study, 23% of Stage I, 38% of Stage II and 50% of Stage III patients had extrinsic cells in the bone marrow (31). Several other investigators have obtained similar results. In the original study from the Ludwig Institute (2), the presence of bone marrow occult metastases was correlated with the tumor stage ($p = 0.05$), and vascular invasion ($p < 0.01$), both of which are known predictors of poor prognosis.

While the presence of bone marrow occult metastases appears to be correlated with known features of disease progression, the ultimate utility of this test will be determined by whether bone marrow occult metastases predict breast cancer recurrence. Several studies now show that, in fact, the presence of occult metastases in the bone marrow identifies a population of patients at high risk for recurrence. Our own studies (6) have revealed that the presence of occult metastases in the bone marrow significantly predicts recurrence; the two-year recurrence rate for patients with no evidence of bone marrow occult metastases was 3% compared with 33% for patients with detectable bone marrow occult metastases. Diel and associates (36) studied 727 patients with primary operable breast cancer. They were able to detect tumor cells in the bone marrow of 203 (55%) of 367 lymph node positive patients and in 112 (31%) of 360 lymph node negative patients. They found that the occult bone marrow metastases were associated with larger tumor size ($p < 0.001$), lymph node involvement ($p = 0.001$) and higher tumor grade ($p = 0.002$). After a median follow-up of 36 months, patients with cancer cells in their bone marrow had reduced disease-free survival times and reduced overall survival (both p values < 0.001). They also found that occult metastases in bone marrow was an independent prognostic indicator for both distant disease-free survival and overall survival that was superior to axillary lymph node status, tumor stage and tumor grade. In a more recent study, Mansi and associates (37) looked at bone marrow aspirates from 350 women with primary breast cancer. In their study, 25% (89/350) were found to have occult metastases by immunohistochemistry. While they found that patients with occult metastases to the bone marrow did have shorter relapse-free and overall survival times, it was not found to be an independent prognostic indicator when tumor size, lymph node status and vascular invasion were taken into account (37). Finally, Braun and associates (38) analyzed the bone marrow samples from 552 patients with Stage I, II or III breast cancer by immunohistochemical methods. They found cytokeratin positive cells in 36% (199/552) of the patients studied. Forty-nine of the 199 (25%) with occult metastases to the bone marrow died of cancer-related causes, while only 49 of 353 (14%) without occult metastases in the bone marrow died ($p < 0.001$). They concluded that the presence of occult metastatic cells in the bone marrow was an independent prognostic indicator of the risk of death from cancer (38).

These large studies provide definitive evidence that the detection of occult metastases by immunohistochemical methods is prognostically important. The presence of bone marrow occult metastases predicts a higher risk for recurrence in bone, as well as in other sites. Of particular importance in all of these findings is the fact that the presence of bone marrow occult metastases identifies patients with node negative disease who are at a higher risk for recurrence; this subset of patients can therefore be the target of more aggressive adjuvant therapy. The studies by both Diel (36) and Braun (38) have shown that bone marrow metastasis is a more powerful predictor of recurrence than histologic node status.

In fact, several studies have now shown that the bone marrow status can be combined with other prognostic factors such as axillary lymph node status. This allows groups of patients to be stratified (6, 16, 36, 39, 40) as follows: (i) those with very low recurrence rates (lymph node negative, bone marrow negative), (ii) those with moderate rates of recurrence (lymph node negative, bone marrow positive, and lymph node positive, bone marrow negative), and (iii) those with high recurrence rates (lymph node positive, bone marrow positive) (6, 36, 40, 41). Diel has suggested that there is consistent evidence that tumor cell detection is a prognostic indicator independent of nodal status and raises the question whether bone marrow aspiration could replace axillary dissection in certain subgroups of patients with clinically negative axilla and tumors less than 2 cm in diameter (36). The prospect of potentially saving a patient from an axillary node dissection is especially attractive when one considers that the morbidity of a bone marrow aspiration is far less than that of an axillary node dissection.

2.2.3 Detection of Bone Marrow Occult Metastases: Effect of Tumor Burden

Another interesting finding from our studies (6) in the detection of occult metastases in the bone marrow is that the number of carcinoma cells detected in the bone marrow (the bone marrow tumor burden) was significantly associated with disease recurrence. In our study, the bone marrow aspirates were processed, so that the concentration of bone marrow elements was equal for each patient. Consequently, the number of extrinsic cells counted for each case could be compared among patients; the number of extrinsic cells identified in the bone marrow was considered to be reflective of the peripheral tumor burden in each patient. Among patients with occult bone marrow metastases, those who did not recur had on average fewer extrinsic cells in their marrow than those who recurred (15 vs. 43 cells respectively). In addition, the estimated 2-year recurrence rate of patients with 10 or more cells (46%) was significantly higher than that of patients with less than 10 cells. Further, the number of extrinsic cells detected in the bone marrow was an independent predictor of prognosis. Braun and associates (38) in their study found that the number of detectable tumor cells (3 per 2×10^6) increased with tumor stage but that exclusion of samples with less than the median number of tumor cells did not change the statistical significance of their findings.

2.3 Detection of Occult Bone Marrow Metastases in Patients with Advanced Breast Carcinoma

Another situation in which detecting occult bone marrow metastases could be of importance is in advanced-stage breast cancer patients who will receive autologous bone marrow transplantation therapy. It is logical to assume that tumor cells in the bone marrow may be re-infused along with the stem cells during such therapy. Whether or not they are a cause of subsequent relapse is not clearly understood. In patients with hematopoietic tumors who have received bone marrow transplantation, disease relapse is thought to result from both re-infusion of tumor cells and re-growth of tumor not killed by systemic treatment. However, in the case of solid tumors, such as breast cancer, the cause of relapse following autologous bone marrow transplantation remains to be determined. Clearly, re-infusion of contaminating tumor cells and re-growth of existent tumor may both play a role. Tumor cells in the bone marrow may be either the cause of relapse or simply a manifestation of tumor deposits outside of bone and, thus, a measure of systemic tumor burden; patients with increased systemic tumor burden may also be at an increased risk for treatment failure. In any event, the presence of bone marrow occult metastases may place patients who will receive autologous bone marrow transplantation at an increased risk for treatment failure and relapse. Several studies (42, 43) examining patients with neuroblastoma and lymphoma suggest that peripheral blood progenitor cell samples may contain fewer tumor cells than does bone marrow. We have shown that the frequency of detecting breast cancer cells in a peripheral blood progenitor cell harvest from patients with localized or metastatic breast cancer is low, even when the bone marrow demonstrates overt or occult disease. While this suggests that bone marrow might be a more suitable site for detecting occult metastases in early-stage breast cancer, it also suggests that peripheral blood may be a more suitable source of progenitor cells for hematopoietic support following high-dose chemotherapy. Peripheral blood has certain other advantages over bone marrow for autologous stem cell transplantation therapy, including the convenience and a faster hematopoeitic recovery.

3 LYMPH NODES

3.1 Detection of Occult Metastases in the Lymph Nodes

Despite the explosion in our knowledge of the biology of cancer, the single most important prognostic factor for most solid tumors is the presence of histologically detectable regional lymph node metastases: patients with tumors that have not metastasized to the regional lymph nodes tend to do far better than patients with lymph node metastases. A significant proportion of node-negative patients will, however, develop distant metastasis. As we have seen, systemic dissemination may take place by routes other than lymphatic spread; the presence of bone marrow occult metastases in node negative patients demonstrates this. Nevertheless, a proportion of node negative patients without the evidence of bone marrow metastases will experience recurrence. It has now become clear that another possible site for occult tumor spread in histologically node negative patients is the regional lymph nodes.

Routine histopathological examination of lymph nodes is, in reality, only a lymph node sampling; in fact, Gusterson and Ott (44) have calculated that a pathologist has only a 1% chance of identifying a metastatic focus of cancer with a diameter of three cells in cross-section occupying a lymph node. It has also been clearly shown that reexamination of lymph node sections initially considered negative for tumor after routine histopathologic screening frequently shows metastatic deposits, demonstrating that even when tumor cells are present in the section, they can be missed (45). It is evident that routine processing and histologic examination of regional lymph nodes is inadequate to detect the presence of tumor in all cases.

Most studies have involved the detection of regional (axillary) lymph node occult metastases in patients with breast cancer (45–52). These studies can be classified into two major categories: (a) detection of metastasis after more intensive histological examination of the lymph node, including analysis of multiple serial sections, and (b) studies which use immunohistochemistry to take advantage of the differential expression of antigens between normal lymph node constituents and epithelial carcinoma cells in order to detect occult tumor in lymph nodes. In fact, this is the same principle as that used for detecting occult tumor in bone marrow. Attempts have also been made to use molecular techniques to detect lymph node occult metastatic cells (52–65).

While studies concerning occult lymph node metastases are most advanced for breast cancer, there is now a growing body of literature on the detection and the clinical significance of occult lymph node metastases in other tumors, such as colon, lung and prostate carcinoma, and melanoma.

3.1.1 Detection of Occult Lymph Node Metastases by Histological Review

Studies undertaken to detect occult lymph node metastases by routine histologic methods have generally been performed by cutting serial sections from all paraffin blocks containing lymph nodes, followed by routine staining and microscopic review (56). However, several studies have simply reviewed again the original histologic slides. All of these studies have demonstrated that deposits of tumor can be detected using these methods. Between 7% and 33% of previously node negative cases convert to node positive after review. As reviewed by Neville (63), the mean conversion rate is approximately 13%.

3.1.2 Detection of Occult Lymph Node Metastases by Immunohistochemistry

Several investigators have used various antibodies in order to detect occult lymph node metastases in patients with breast cancer using immunohistochemical methods. In general, most studies have used antibodies specific for low molecular weight intermediate filament proteins to distinguish the epithelial tumor deposits from normal node elements. Other studies have used antimucin antibodies raised against human mammary carcinoma cells (62). In our own studies, we have used a cocktail of two antikeratin antibodies, AE1 and CAM5.2 (which in combination recognize cytokeratin 18 and 19, the predominant intermediate filament proteins in simple epithelial cells). While antibodies to cytokeratins have been reported to react with dendritic reticulum cells (with the possibility of producing false positive results), this has not been a significant problem in our own experiments. Furthermore, as with the bone marrow examination previously described, the morphologic evaluation of the 'positive' cells is critical; cells that do not possess the morphologic characteristics of malignant epithelial cells are not considered tumor cells in our studies.

Unlike routine histological evaluation for the detection of occult metastases in which multiple sections from each block are studied, most of the studies employing immunohistochemical techniques have tested only a single section. When a single section is studied, the percentage of patients who convert from node negative to node positive ranges from 14% to 30% with a mean conversion rate of 16%, as reviewed by Neville (45, 63).

3.1.3 Detection of Occult Lymph Node Metastases by RT-PCR

While it may at some point be possible to detect occult metastases in the lymph nodes of patients with breast cancer using PCR methods, this procedure continues to have major drawbacks compared with immunohistochemistry. In addition to the problems of identifying appropriately sensitive and specific markers discussed above, the lymph nodes used must be fresh (or fresh frozen), and traditionally all lymph nodes in their entirety must be disaggregated to undergo RNA extraction (as we have shown that metastases in node negative cases usually occurs to only one lymph node). Therefore, these lymph nodes will be totally unavailable for histologic review, and the method will test for both histologic and occult positives. However, new techniques such as laser capture microdissection will allow frozen sections of lymph nodes to be analyzed for morphologic evidence of tumor and the individual tumor cells can be dissected for RT-PCR analysis. This is in contrast to immunohistochemical techniques, which can be done on formalin-fixed, paraffin-embedded tissue that has been routinely prepared for histologic evaluation.

3.2 Clinical Significance of Occult Lymph Node Metastases in Patients with Breast Cancer

Although virtually all studies have demonstrated that lymph node metastases can be overlooked, there is a surprising disagreement about the prognostic importance of these occult tumor deposits. Many of the studies using routine histologic review of sections have found that the presence of occult lymph node metastases does not influence the recurrence rates in a statistically significant way (47–49); several studies using immunohistochemical techniques have reported similar findings (53, 54, 60). In order to begin to understand this, a few basic observations need to be made. Many earlier studies have involved fewer than 100 patients; in fact, some have involved even fewer than 50 patients. Cote and Groshen have demonstrated that even if the finding of occult lymph node metastases is prognostically important, there is no possibility that studies of the clinical impact of occult lymph node metastases involving few patients will provide statistically significant data (unpublished data). In fact, Fisher *et al.* (48) were the first to clearly point this out: ‘it has been mathematically estimated that differences in survival of 10 percent, if indeed they occur between the two groups [true lymph node negative versus occult lymph node positive], would require a study of approximately 1400 cases.’ Therefore, studies involving a few patients are not suitable to address the issue of prognostic significance of occult lymph node metastases.

Fortunately, investigators from the Ludwig Institute and International Breast Cancer study group have performed a definitive study of the importance of occult lymph node metastases in patients with node negative breast cancer (50). They examined serial sections of 921 node negative breast cancer patients by routine histological methods. Nine percent of these patients were found to have occult lymph node metastases; these patients had a poorer disease-free ($p = 0.003$) and overall survival ($p = 0.002$) after 5 years' median follow-up, compared with patients whose nodes remained negative after serial sectioning. Six-year median follow-up data give even more conclusive evidence of the prognostic significance of occult lymph node metastases. Another large-scale study was performed by de Mascarel *et al.* (51), with a median follow-up of 7 years. These investigators studied the lymph nodes from 1,121 patients with primary operable breast cancer, by serial macroscopic sectioning; they found single occult lymph node metastases in 120 patients. A significant difference in recurrence ($p = 0.005$) and survival ($p = 0.04$) was found between node negative patients and those with single occult metastases. However, in multivariate analysis using the Cox model, occult metastases were not a predicting factor. Several studies using immunohistochemical methods have also shown the prognostic significance of occult lymph node metastases (55, 57, 62). In a more recent study, we examined the lymph nodes from 736 patients with breast cancer who were involved in Trial V of the International (Ludwig) Breast Cancer Study for the presence of metastases. Occult metastases were detected by immunohistochemistry in

148 (20%) of 736 patients. These occult metastases were associated with significantly poor disease-free and overall survival in postmenopausal patients but not in premenopausal patients. Immunohistochemically detected occult lymph node metastases remained an independent and highly significant predictor of recurrence, even after control for tumor grade, tumor size, estrogen-receptor status, vascular invasion and treatment ($p = 0.007$) (66).

While there is ample evidence showing that occult lymph node metastases can be detected in a substantial proportion of node negative patients and that the presence of such deposits is probably prognostically significant, the best method for detecting these deposits is not yet clear. Re-examination of multiple serial sections is laborious, time-consuming and expensive. Immunohistochemical assays, on the other hand, are more sensitive and certainly less laborious. Definitive comparative analyses are now ongoing; results from these studies suggest that immunohistochemical methods may be superior to histologic re-examination of lymph node serial sections (66).

3.3 Sentinel Lymph Nodes

Axillary lymph node dissection (ALND) has been the standard in care for patients with breast cancer. In more recent years, the sentinel lymph node dissection (SLND) technique has been extensively studied. The technique uses isosulfan blue dye, a radiopharmaceutical, or a combination of both to locate and remove the first few lymph nodes that drain the tumor. These sentinel lymph nodes are considered the most likely to contain cancer cells. This procedure has the advantage of potentially saving patients with early-stage breast cancer from having a complete axillary lymph node dissection and the subsequent morbidity that is associated with this procedure. Several studies have shown that this technique is highly accurate in staging patients. Giuliano *et al.* (67) showed a false-negative rate for patients who had an ALND performed after SLND of only 2%. Veronesi *et al.* (68) reported no false-negative sentinel lymph nodes among 45 patients with T1 breast cancer that measured less than 1.5 cm. The overall accuracy rate that included T3 tumors was 97%. Furthermore, Alex and Krag (69) were able to identify the sentinel lymph nodes in 50 of the 70 patients they studied. Of these 50 patients, 18 were found to have positive sentinel nodes that were predictive of the axillary status. Albertini *et al.* (70) were able to identify the sentinel lymph nodes in 57 of 62 (92%) patients. All patients with axillary nodal metastases were identified by the sentinel lymph node examination. However, a trial that looked at the sentinel lymph nodes from multiple institutions using only the radioisotope technique alone showed somewhat less promising results (71). In this study of 443 patients, a sentinel lymph node was identified in 405 patients. These 405 then underwent a completion axillary lymph node dissection. Of these 405, there were 114 node positive cases with 13 false negative nodes for a false negative rate of 11%.

In cases in which the routine histologic examination of the sentinel lymph node is negative, immunohistochemical evaluation for the presence of occult metastases may play an important role in the histopathologic evaluation of these patients. The reported rate of positivity for occult metastases in these hiostologically negative nodes ranges from 5% to 15% (72). It is clear that large-scale clinical trials are needed to determine the clinical relevance of these occult metastases positive sentinel lymph nodes.

4 FUTURE DIRECTIONS

The true test of the prognostic importance of occult metastasis detection in both the bone marrow and lymph nodes will come from large-scale multi-institutional studies. In the case of breast cancer, such a study is now well under way, under the auspices of the American College of Surgeons Oncology Group (ACOSOG), protocol Z0010 'A prognostic study of sentinel node and bone marrow micrometastases in women with clinical T1-2 N0 breast cancer'. This study should provide definitive evidence of the prognostic significance of occult metastases in patients with breast cancer.*

We have suggested a new concept in the staging of cancers using the TNM classification, where the traditional T (tumor), N (node) and M (metastasis) may be complemented by *n* and *m* (nodal and systemic occult metastases); that is, TN*n*M*m* (73, 74). With the results of larger studies on prognostic significance of occult metastases, either in bone marrow or lymph nodes, this staging may be applied clinically. The estimates of outcome for populations of patients may be narrowed down to those for sub-populations of patients (i.e., those with or without occult metastases). Similarly, in future, treatment decisions may be based on the detection of occult metastases.

*Funded by RO1 CA 85840-01

REFERENCES

1. Schabel FM. Rationalc for adjuvant chcmothcrapy. Cancer. 1977; 39: 2875–2882.
2. Redding WH, Monaghan P, Imrie SF. Detection of micrometastases in patients with primary breast cancer. Lancet. 1982: 1271–1274.
3. Osborne MP, Asina S, Wong GY. Immunofluorescent monoclonal antibody detection of breast cancer in bone marrow: sensitivity in a model system. Cancer Res. 1989; 49: 2510.
4. Osborne MP, Wong GY, Asina S. Sensitivity of immunocytochemical detection of breast cancer cells in human bone marrow. Cancer Res. 1991; 51: 2706.
5. Ellis G, Fergusson M, Yamanaka E. Monoclonal antibodies for detection of occult carcinoma cells in bone marrow of breast cancer patients. Cancer. 1989; 63: 2509–2514.
6. Cote RJ, Rosen PP, Lesser ML, Old LJ, Osborne MP. Prediction of early relapse in patients with operable breast cancer by detection of occult bone marrow micrometastases. J. Clin. Oncol. 1991; 9: 1749–1756.
7. Schlimok G, Funke I, Bock B, Witte J, Riethmuller G. Epithelial tumor cells in bone marrow of patients with colorectal cancer: immunocytochemical detection, phenotypic characterization, and prognostic significance. J. Clin. Oncol. 1990; 8: 831–837.

8. Lindeman F, Schlimok G, Dirschedl P, Witte J, Riethmuller G. Prognostic significance of micrometastatic tumor cells in bone marrow of colorectal cancer patients. Lancet. 1992; 340: 685–689.
9. Silly H, Samanigg H, Stoger H, Brezinschek HP, Wilders-Trusching M. Micrometastatic tumor cells in bone marrow in colorectal carcinoma. Lancet. 1992; 340: 1288.
10. Moreno JG, Croce CM, Fischer R *et al.* Detection of hematogenous micrometastases in patients with prostate cancer. Cancer Res. 1992; 52: 6110–6112.
11. Oberneder R, Riesenberg R, Kriegmair M *et al.* Immunocytochemical detection and phenotypic characterization of micrometastatic tumour cells in bone marrow of patients with prostate cancer. Urol. Res. 1994; 22: 3–8.
12. Bretton PR, Melamed MR, Fair WR, Cote RJ. Detection of occult micrometastases in the bone marrow of patients with prostate carcinoma. Prostate. 1994; 25: 108–114.
13. Wood DPJ, Banks ER, Humphreys S *et al.* Identification of bone marrow micrometastases in patients with prostate cancer. Cancer. 1994; 74: 2533–2540.
14. Frew AJ, Ralkaier N, Ghosh AK, Gatter KC, Mason DY. Immunohistochemistry in the detection of bone marrow micrometastases in patients with primary lung cancer. Brit. J. Cancer. 1986; 53: 555–556.
15. Leonard RCF, Duncan LW, Hay FG. Immunocytological detection of residual marrow disease at clinical remission predicts metastatic relapse in small cell lung cancer. Cancer Res. 1990; 50: 6545–6548.
16. Pantel K, Izbicki JR, Angswurm M *et al.* Immunocytological detection of bone marrow micrometastasis in operable non-small cell lung cancer. Cancer Res. 1993; 53(5): 1027–1031.
17. Pantel K, Isbicki J, Passlick B *et al.* Frequency and prognostic significance of isolated tumour cells in bone marrow of patients with non-small cell lung cancer without overt metastases. Lancet. 1996; 347: 649–653.
18. Cote RJ, Beattie EJ, Chaiwun B *et al.* Detection of occult bone marrow metastases in patients with operable lung carcinoma. Ann. Surg. 1995; 222: 415–425.
19. Datta YH, Adams PT, Drobski WR *et al.* Sensitive detection of occult breast cancer by reverse-transcriptase polymerase chain reaction. J. Clin. Oncol. 1994; 12: 475–482.
20. Bostick PJ, Chatterjee S, Chi DD *et al.* Limitations of specific reverse-transcriptase polymerase chain reaction markers in the detection of metastases in the lymph nodes and blood of breast cancer patients. J. Clin. Oncol. 1998; 16: 2632–2640.
21. Zippelius P, Kufer P, Honold G *et al.* Limitations of reverse-transcriptase polymerase chain reaction analysis for detection of micrometastatic epithelial cancer cells in bone marrow. J. Clin. Oncol. 1997; 15: 2701–2708.
22. Grunewald K, Haun M, Urbanek M *et al.* Mammoglobin gene expression; a superior marker of breast cancer cells in peripheral blood in comparison to epidermal-growth-factor receptor and cytokeratin-19. Laboratory Investigations. 2000; 80: 1071–1077.
23. Watson MA, Dintzis S, Darrow CM *et al.* Mammoglobin expression in primary, metastatic, and occult breast cancer. Cancer Res. 1999; 59: 3028–3031.
24. Zach O, Kasparu H, Kriegar O *et al.* Detection of circulating mammary carcinoma cells in the peripheral blood of breast cancer patients via nested reverse transcriptase polymerase chain reaction assay for mammoglobin mRNA. J. Clin. Oncol. 1999; 17: 2015–2019.
25. Gross HJ, Verwer B, Houck D, Hoffman RA, Recketenwald D. Model study detecting breast cancer cells in peripheral blood mononuclear cells at frequencies as low as 10-7. Proc. Natl. Acad. Sci. USA. 1995; 92: 537–541.

26. Leslie DS, Johnston WW, Daly L *et al.* Detection of breast carcinoma cells in human bone marrow using fluorescent-activated cell sorting and conventional cytology. Am. J. Clin. Pathol. 1990; 94: 8–13.
27. Kim SJ, Ikeda N, Shiba E, Takamura Y, Noguchi S. Detection of breast cancer micrometastases in peripheral blood using immunomagnetic separation and immunocytochemistry. Breast Cancer. 2001; 8: 63–69.
28. Slade MJ, Smith BM, Sinnett D, Cross NCP, Coombes RC. Quantitiative polymerase chain reaction for the detection of micrometastases in patients with breast cancer. J. Clin. Oncology. 1999; 17: 870–879.
29. Theriult RL, Hortobagy GN. Bone metastases in breast cancer. Anticancer Drugs. 1992; 3: 455–462.
30. Body JJ. Metastatic bone disease: clinical and therapeutic aspects. Bone. 1992; 13(Suppl.): 857–862.
31. Cote RJ, Rosen PP, Hakes TB *et al.* Monoclonal antibodies detect occult breast carcinoma metastases in bone marrow of patients with early-stage disease. Am. J. Surg. Pathol. 1988; 12: 333.
32. Berger U, Bettelheim R, Mansi JL, Easton D, Coombes RC, Neville AM. The relationship between micrometastases in the bone marrow, histopathologic features in the primary tumor in breast cancer and prognosis. Am. J. Clin. Pathol. 1988; 90: 1–6.
33. Osborne MP, Rosen PP. Detection and management of bone marrow micrometastases in breast cancer. Oncology (Huntingt). 1994; 8: 25–31.
34. Mansi JL, Berger U, Easton D *et al.* Micrometastases in bone marrow in patients with primary breast cancer: evaluation as an early predictor of bone metastases. Br. Med. J. 1987; 295: 1093–1096.
35. Porro G, Ménard S, Tagliabue E *et al.* Monoclonal antibody detection of carcinoma cells in bone marrow biopsy specimens from breast cancer patients. Cancer. 1988; 61: 2407.
36. Diel IJ, Kaufmann M, Costa SD *et al.* Micrometastatic breast cancer cells in bone marrow at primary surgery: prognostic value in comparison with nodal status. J. Natl. Cancer Inst. 1997; 88: 1652–1658.
37. Mansi JL, Gogas H, Bliss JM, Gazet J-C, Berger U, Coombes RC. Outcome of primary-breast-cancer patients with micrometastases: a long-term follow-up study. Lancet. 1999; 354: 197–202.
38. Braun S, Pantel K, Muller P *et al.* Cytokeratin-positive cells in the bone marrow and survival of patients with stage I, II, or III breast cancer. N. Eng. J. Med. 2000; 342: 525–533.
39. Dearnaley DP, Ormerod MG, Sloane JP. Micrometastases in breast cancer: long-term follow-up of the first patient cohort. Eur. J. Cancer. 1991; 27: 236.
40. Mansi JL, Easton U, Berger JC *et al.* Bone marrow micrometastases in primary breast cancer: prognostic significance after six years' follow-up. Eur. J. Cancer. 1991; 27: 1552.
41. Diel IJ, Kaufman M, Goener R *et al.* Detection of tumor cells in bone marrow of patients with primary breast cancer: a prognostic factor for distant metastases. J. Clin. Oncol. 1992; 10: 1534–1539.
42. Kessinger A, Armitage JO, Smith DM *et al.* High-dose therapy and autologous peripheral blood stem cell transplantation for patients with lymphoma. Blood. 1989; 74: 1260–1265.
43. Moss TJ, Reynolds CP, Sather SN *et al.* Prognostic value of immunohistochemical detection of bone marrow metastases in neuroblastoma. N. Eng. J. Med. 1991; 324: 219–226.

44. Gusterson BA, Ott R. Occult axillary lymph node micrometastases in breast cancer. Lancet. 1990; 336: 434–435.
45. Neville AM. Breast cancer micrometastases in lymph nodes and bone marrow are prognostically important. Ann. Oncol. 1989; 2: 13–14.
46. Saphir O, Amromin GD. Obscurc axillary lymph node metastases in carcinoma of the breast. Cancer. 1948; 1: 238–241.
47. Pickren JW. Significance of occult metastases. A study of breast cancer. Cancer. 1961; 14: 1266–1271.
48. Fisher ER, Saminoss S, Lee CH *et al.* Detection and significance of occult axillary node metastases in patients with invasive breast cancer. Cancer. 1978; 42: 2025–2031.
49. Wilkinson EJ, Hause LL, Hoffman RG *et al.* Occult axillary lymph node metastases in invasive breast carcinoma: characteristics of the primary tumor and the significance of metastases. Pathol. Ann. 1982; 17: 67–91.
50. International (LUDWIG) Breast Cancer Study Group. Prognostic importance of occult lymph node micrometastases from breast cancers. Lancet. 1990; 335: 1565–1568.
51. de Mascarel I, Bonichon F, Coindre JM, Trojani M. Prognostic significance of breast cancer axillary lymph node micrometastases assessed by two special techniques: reevaluation with longer follow-up. Brit. J. Cancer. 1992; 66: 523–527.
52. Wells CA, Heryt A, Brochier J *et al.* The immunohistochemical detection of axillary micrometastases in breast cancer. Brit. J. Cancer. 1984; 50: 193–197.
53. Bussolati G, Gugliotta P, Morra Z *et al.* The immunohistochemical detection of lymph node micrometastases from infiltrating lobular carcinoma of the breast. Brit. J. Cancer. 1986; 54: 631–636.
54. Byrne J, Waldron R, McAvinchy D *et al.* The use of monoclonal antibodies for the histological detection of mammary axillary micrometastases. Eur. J. Surg. Oncol. 1987; 13: 409.
55. Trojani L, de Mascarel I, Bonichon F *et al.* Micrometastases to axillary lymph nodes from carcinoma of the breast: detection by immunohistochemistry and prognostic significance. Brit. J. Cancer. 1987; 55: 303–306.
56. Apostolikas N, Petraki C, Agnantis NJ. The reliability of histologically negative axillary lymph nodes in breast cancer. Pathol. Res. Pract. 1989; 184: 35–38.
57. Sedmak DD, Meinke TA, Knechtges DS *et al.* Prognostic significance of cytokeratin-positive breast cancer metastases. Mod. Pathol. 1989; 2: 516–520.
58. Cote RJ, Chaiwun B, Qu J, Agnantis NJ *et al.* Prognostic importance of occult lymph node metastases in patients with breast cancer. Proc. Am. Assoc. Cancer Res. 1992; 33: 202.
59. Neville AM, Price KN, Gelber RD *et al.* Axillary lymph node micrometastases and breast cancer. Lancet. 1991; 337: 110.
60. Elson CE, Kufe D, Johnston WW. Immunohistochemical detection and significance of axillary lymph node micrometastases in breast cancer – a study of 97 cases. Anal. Quant. Cytol. Histol. 1993: 171–178.
61. Nasser IA, Lee AKC, Bosari S, Saganich R, Heatly G, Silverman ML. Occult axillary lymph node metastases in 'node-negative' breast cancer. Hum. Pathol. 1993; 24: 950–957.
62. Hainsworth PJ, Tjandra JJ, Stillwell RG *et al.* Detection and significance of occult metastases in node-negative breast cancer. Brit. J. Surg. 1993; 80: 459–463.
63. Neville AM. Prognostic factors and primary breast cancer. Diag. Oncol. 1991; 1: 53.
64. Schoenfeld A, Luqmani Y, Smith D *et al.* Detection of breast cancer micrometastases in axillary nodes using polymerase chain reaction. Cancer Res. 1994; 54: 2986–2990.

65. Noguchi S, Aihara T, Nakamori S *et al.* The detection of breast cancer micrometastases in axillary lymph nodes by means of reverse-transcriptase polymerase chain reaction. Cancer. 1994; 74: 1595–1600.
66. Cote RJ, Peterson HF, Chaiwun B *et al.* Role of immunohistochemical detection of lymph-node metastases in management of breast cancer. Lancet. 1999; 354: 896–900.
67. Giuliano AE, Jones RC, Brennan M, Statman R. Sentinel lymphadenectomy in breast cancer. J. Clin. Oncol. 1997; 15: 2345.
68. Veronesi U, Paganelli G, Galimberti V *et al.* Sentinel-node biopsy to avoid axillary dissection in breast cancer with clinically negative lymph-nodes. Lancet. 1997; 349: 1864–1867.
69. Alex JC, Krag DN. The gamma-probe-guided resection of radiolabeled primary lymph nodes. Surg. Oncol. Clin. N. Am. 1996; 5: 33–41.
70. Albertini JJ, Lyman GH, Cox C *et al.* Lymphatic mapping and sentinel node biopsy in the patient with breast cancer. JAMA. 1996; 276: 1818–1822.
71. Krag DN, Weaver D, Ashikaga T *et al.* The sentinel node in breast cancer: a multicenter validation study. N. Eng. J. Med. 1998; 339(14): 941–995.
72. Turner RR, Ollila DW, Krasne DL, Giuliano AE. Histopathologic validation of the sentinel lymph node hypothesis for breast carcinoma. Ann. Surg. 1997; 226: 271–278.
73. Cote RJ, Hawes D, Chaiwun B, Beattie EJ. Detection of occult metastases in lung carcinomas: progress and implications for staging. J. Surg. Oncol. 1998; 69: 265–274.
74. Chaiwun B, Saad A, Chatterjee SJ, Taylor CR, Beattie EJ, Cote RJ. Advances in the pathologic staging of lung cancer: detection of regional and systemic occult metastases. In: Marchevsky AM, Koss MN, eds. State of the Art Reviews. Philadelphia: Hanley & Belfus, 1996, pp. 155–168.

Chapter 5

DETECTION, ISOLATION AND STUDY OF DISSEMINATED PROSTATE CANCER CELLS IN THE PERIPHERAL BLOOD AND BONE MARROW

Jesco Pfitzenmaier, Robert L. Vessella, William J. Ellis, Paul H. Lange

Department of Urology, University of Washington Medical School, Seattle, USA

Abstract

About 20% to 40% of men who undergo a radical prostatectomy for localized prostate cancer will relapse with progressive disease that frequently results in bone metastases. In addition to numerous studies of the primary tumour, there has been increased attention paid to disseminated cells shed by the tumour and detected in the peripheral blood and bone marrow. It would appear logical that the prostate cancer cells in the blood and the bone marrow that remain following a radical prostatectomy may be more informative in revealing prognostic information than those of the primary tumour which is removed at surgery. The evidence for existence of these disseminated cells in the peripheral blood and bone marrow of prostate cancer patients was first described in the early 1990s using a prostate specific antigen reverse transcriptase polymerase chain reaction (PSA RT-PCR). In general, these studies revealed the presence of disseminated PSA+ epithelial cells (presumed to be prostate cancer cells) early in the disease course and more prevalent in advanced disease than in early disease. Most showed that the bone marrow was more frequently positive than the peripheral blood. As a staging tool, these studies generally showed that PSA RT-PCR was not highly informative since even patients with low stage and early disease frequently showed evidence of disseminated PSA+ cells. Over the past few years, there has been a rapid development of technologies for isolating these disseminated cells for further study. The first step was the enrichment of circulating tumour cells, followed by attempts to isolate and characterize individual cells. The enriched cells have been analysed by a variety of methods, including flow cytometry, immunohistochemistry, and fluorescent *in situ* hybridisation. Biological characterisation of the cells have included the assessment of telomerase activity, androgen receptor status, and genomic alterations such as loss of heterozygosity and microsatellite instability. Attempts are under way to extend this analysis by utilizing gene expression micro-arrays and array Comparative Genomic Hybridisation (array-CGH). Although these efforts encompass challenges much will be learned about the character of these disseminated cells, including their process of trafficking to distant sites, their potential to seed and grow at these sites and their tendencies for cell dormancy.

K. Pantel (ed.), Micrometastasis, 87–116.

INTRODUCTION

Prostate Cancer

Epidemiology and Clinic

In 2001, approximately 198,000 men in the United States were diagnosed with prostate cancer, and nearly 32,000 died from this disease (1, 2). The incidence and possibly mortality has decreased, in part because of early detection efforts. Thus, in 1997, the incidence was 334,500 and the number of deaths caused by this disease was reported as 41,800 (3, 4). Among men in the industrialized countries prostate cancer is the most common cancer diagnosed and represents the second leading cause of death in male cancer patients. Over 90% of prostate cancer is diagnosed in patients between the ages of 45 and 89 years, with a median age of diagnosis of 72 years (5). The incidence rises dramatically with age. As breast cancer, prostate cancer is hormone dependent and people with a positive family history have a higher risk of developing this tumour at a younger age than patients with a negative family history. Incidence and mortality rates are considerably higher among African Americans compared to Caucasians, Asians, and Native Americans (2). The alternatives for treating a patient with localized prostate cancer are many: first, there is the watch and wait strategy that is most relevant for an older patient or a patient with a low Gleason score on biopsy that suggests a less aggressive tumour. The second and most common treatment is the radical prostatectomy (6–8) which can be performed retropubically or perineally. In many circumstances, the nerves controlling potency can be preserved. A third surgical option that is gaining acceptance for removal of the tumorous prostate is laparoscopy (9–12). For those patients who wish treatment but surgical intervention is not desired or is not an option, there is radiation therapy. External beam radiation therapy (13) is one of the two options. The second one is brachytherapy (13, 14) where the prostate gland is implanted with radioactive seeds.

The five-year survival rate for patients with a locally confined prostate cancer is 99% (4), whereas it is 93% for patients with regionally spread cancer (3). Unfortunately, even after therapy for apparently organ-confined disease, 20% to 40% of the patients have the chance of developing biochemical recurrence from persistent disease. While the clinical course of patients with elevated PSA levels are quite variable with some very long intervals between PSA elevation and clinical symptoms, eventually all of these patients will develop bone metastases if they live long enough. One key question is whether the metastases come from pre-existing micrometastases or from persistent disease remaining locally. Then, as in other kinds of malignancy, the five-year survival for a patient with distant metastases is poor, approximately 30% (3) and 0% after ten years. The palliative treatment of a patient with metastatic disease is mainly androgen ablative therapy, allowing the patient to lead a normal life with good results over several years. Because overall up to a third of the patients diagnosed with prostate cancer will develop metastatic disease mainly to the bone, it is important to improve the diagnostic accuracy for early metastatic disease. Unfortunately, even with an early diagnosis of micrometastatic disease, there are no therapies proven to be effective. Hopefully, the further study of disseminated cells will reveal biological and molecular targets that will ultimately change this scenario.

Disseminated Cells in Prostate Cancer

Tumour progression in prostate cancer following radical prostatectomy occurs in 20% to 40% of patients. Even though pathological stage, Gleason score, surgical margin status, and PSA levels are useful prognosticators, the prediction of whether an individual patient will relapse years later with progressive disease is an inexact science. While there have been numerous attempts to add prognostic power from other biological features gleaned from the resected tumour, including ploidy (15, 16), aneusomy (17, 18), expression of metalloproteinases and many more, none has proven repeatedly to be of higher predictive value than Gleason score (19).

Since dissemination of cancer cells from the primary to distant sites is a prerequisite for metastases, the study of these disseminated cells has been the objective of many investigations. These endeavours have taken on two primary forms. The most classic has been the histological examination of disseminated cells in the blood and in the bone marrow using immunohistological and cytogenetic techniques (20–24). A second approach gained considerable popularity beginning in the early 1990s when investigators hypothesized that the detection of disseminated PSA positive cells in the blood and in the bone marrow by the molecular technique of reverse transcriptase polymerase chain reaction (RT-PCR) at the time of the diagnosis would be a good prognosticator of eventual prostate cancer progression (25–33). The microscopic scrutiny of disseminated prostate cancer cells by immunohistochemistry and cytogenetic techniques, as well as by several molecular approaches, has revealed important information regarding these cells and hints that characteristics will emerge from additional research that will be useful in prognosis of recurrence risk. Detecting the presence of these cells is only the very first step.

Therapy Monitoring and Drug Targeting

In addition to using RT-PCR for the detection of disseminated cells prior to radical prostatectomy, it has also been used to assess the effectiveness of the therapy. In one study (34), PSA RT-PCR had good sensitivity and specificity; it was only positive in 3% of patients without any signs for recurrent disease, whereas the result was positive in 47% of patients with treatment failure showing a significant relation between RT-PCR results and concomitant serum PSA levels. Su *et al.* (35) used prostate-specific membrane antigen (PSMA) as the transcript target for RT-PCR detection of circulating prostate cancer cells preoperatively and postoperatively in 38 pT2 and pT3 prostate cancer patients. They showed a reduction of disseminated cells in the group with antiandrogen treatment and a postoperative increase of circulating cells, probably due to surgical manipulation of the prostate. A third study showed a 75% positivity in blood samples of patients that failed surgical treatment or with metastatic disease (36). Most of the patients who had disseminated cells preoperatively became negative for PSA RT-PCR after the operation. Despite these data, this test could neither be used preoperatively to determine pathological stage nor to predict a treatment failure. Pantel *et al.* (24) used an immunocytochemical approach to show a decrease in cytokeratin 18 positive cells in the bone marrow of 36 Stage C prostate cancer patients before and after androgen ablation treatment with flutamide and leuprorelin acetate. All 7 patients remaining positive after the therapy had non-detectable serum PSA levels despite the findings of disseminated prostate cancer cells in the bone marrow. This is not contradictory as it reaffirms that micrometastatic disease can exist with serum PSA levels being below the level of detection. Further long-term follow-up studies will determine whether these detected cells will develop into clinically relevant metastases or if they are dormant and become of no clinical consequence. At this point, there is no way to differentiate between these cell types using current assays. In another study, Bianco *et al.* (37) showed that the disease-free survival in a group of 58 patients with localized prostate cancer was significantly less when the patients had proliferating cytokeratin-positive cells in their bone marrow.

The molecular characterization of these disseminated cells may provide more information about metastatic potential, drug sensitivity and ability to develop drug resistance than analyses of the primary tumour that is removed during initial treatment. Also, these investigations might reveal subgroups of cancer patients who would benefit from certain therapy protocols based on the characteristics of the disseminated cells. When the initial treatment was removal of the prostate by radical prostatectomy or destruction of the organ and the cancer by external or internal radiation therapy, the disseminated prostate cancer cells represent the residual target for further treatment. The discovery of therapeutic targets on these cells should arise from their comprehensive characterization. There are many who believe that prostate cancer is nearly ideal as a target for cellular immunotherapy or monoclonal antibody therapy and several clinical trials are under way. For example, Boynton *et al.* (38) showed that autologous dendritic cells carrying PSMA peptides may be administered safely to patients and reported a response rate in patients with hormone refractory metastatic disease of 34%. Bander and colleagues have reported considerable promise in early clinical trials (39) where they targeted an external epitope of PSMA with monoclonal antibodies. Similarly, a phase I clinical trial in patients with hormone refractory prostate cancer is under way using an antibody that targets the epidermal growth factor receptor. Schwab *et al.* demonstrated the approach was highly effective in the eradication of established A431 tumours that highly express this receptor (38).

SAMPLE PREPARATION AND METHODS OF DETECTION

Preparing the Sample for Analysis

Regardless of the method used for the detection of disseminated tumour cells in the peripheral blood or bone marrow, the initial step upon receiving the specimen is typically separation of the mononuclear cells and disseminated tumour cells from the other cells in the specimen. The standard procedure utilizes density gradient centrifugation to isolate cells based on their buoyant density. Ficoll-Hypaque (40, 41), as a commonly used gradient, consists of a defined molecular weight polysaccharide and sodium diatrizoate, an iodinated non-ionic compound, the combination of which results in a solution with a density of 1.077 g/ml. It is used to separate the red blood cells and granulocytes that have densities >1.077 g/ml from the mononuclear cells (MNC) that have a density <1.077 g/ml. Following centrifugation of the specimen from normal subjects, the interphase between the specimen and the Ficoll-Hypaque solution consists of the MNC. Using peripheral blood or bone marrow specimens from cancer patients, the interphase may also contain disseminated epithelial tumour cells. This interphase can be used for direct investigation (e.g., cytology, RT-PCR, immunohistology) or can be further processed for enrichment of the tumour cells (see section on enrichment). Other media similar to Ficoll-Hypaque that are used to separate cells by density gradient centrifugation are OncoQuick, LymphoPrep, Ficoll-Paque, PolymorphPrep and NycoPrep (42). As shown by Wang *et al.* (43), one can also use two different density gradients (1.068 g/ml and 1.083 g/ml) to achieve a higher purification of the mononuclear cell layer.

Immunohistochemistry and Immunophenotyping

The first steps to identify circulating tumour cells in blood or bone marrow specimens were undertaken in the late 1980s by using immunohistochemical approaches. Several studies showed that immunocytochemistry was superior to conventional cytology or histology for the detection of disseminated tumour cells (44, 45). Many studies followed in the early 1990s as monoclonal antibodies became more prevalent (20, 22, 46–48). Subsequently, immunohistochemical detection of disseminated cells was supplemented by additional cytogenetic techniques that added information regarding the proliferative status and numerical abnormalities of chromosomes (49, 50). The target antigen for immunohistochemical detection and immunophenotyping of disseminated cells is often a protein expressed on the plasma membrane. One common surface marker in prostate cancer cells is PSMA (51). Cytoplasmic markers, such as PSA, may also be targets but this necessitates the permeabilization of the cell, so that the antibody has access to the protein.

Although simple in concept, the detection of disseminated prostate cancer cells by immunohistology has yielded variable results. Bretton *et al.* (20) used a panel of three monoclonal antibodies directed against cytoskeletal and membrane antigens to detect tumour cells in bone marrow aspirates from 20 prostate cancer patients. They found 22% of patients with localized cancer positive for epithelial cells in their bone marrow, whereas metastatic prostate cancer patients showed a positivity rate of 36%. The serum PSA level of patients with localized cancer and positive bone marrow cells was 26.6 ng/ml compared to 12.3 ng/ml in patients without disseminated cells. Mueller *et al.* (49) identified epithelial cells in bone marrow aspirates using an antibody that reacted with cytokeratins 8 and 18 and further examined proliferation status by looking at the expression of proliferating cell nuclear antigen (PCNA) and PSA. They found that approximately 45% of these patients had cytokeratin positive cells in their aspirates. None was PCNA positive, and a few (12%) were PSA positive. The frequency of detection of cytokeratin positive cells was similar to that of previous studies (22, 46, 52). For example, Oberneder *et al.* (46) were able to detect isolated prostate tumour cells in 33% of 84 patients with tumour stage N0M0. Furthermore, they showed a correlation with established risk factors such as local tumour extent, distant metastases and tumour differentiation. Similarly, using an anti-cytokeratin 18 (CK 18) monoclonal antibody, Pantel *et al.* (22) reported that 54.5% of 44 patients with Stage C prostate cancer had CK 18 expressing cells. In contrast to the aforementioned series, Weckermann *et al.* (53) reported a 23.7% positivity rate for CK 18 expressing cells in preoperatively removed bone marrow aspirates of 287 prostate cancer patients and found no correlation to other risk factors such as Gleason score, pathologic stage, ploidy, and preoperative serum prostate specific antigen level. With a median follow-up of 32 months, they were not able to demonstrate a significantly earlier biochemical relapse in 169 patients with localized prostate cancer, comparing patients with and without CK 18 expressing cells in their preoperative bone marrow aspirates (54). In contrast, patients who had disseminated cells in their preoperative bone marrow, as determined using a pan-cytokeratin antibody that recognized a common epitope of cytokeratin 8, 18 and 19, had a significantly earlier biochemical progression than those patients without positive cells preoperatively (55).

Flow Cytometry

By the end of the 1980s, the application of flow cytometry to the assessment and separation of heterogeneous cell populations added additional clout to the analysis of tumour cells. With this technique, a methodology was available to analyse hundreds of cells per second and perform several measurements to be made simultaneously on the same cell. The first studies published were primarily focused on the flow cytometric assessment of tumour ploidy (15, 56, 57). With further development of this technique during the 1990s, flow cytometry was used to detect surface antigens on prostate cancer cells as shown by our colleagues

Liu *et al.* (58–60). These studies showed that the $CD57^+$ cancer cell type predominated in primary tumours, whereas $CD44^+$ cancer cells were predominant in visceral metastases of prostate cancer. In addition to these investigations, flow cytometry was being used more frequently to detect and sort disseminated prostate cancer cells in blood and bone marrow samples. Flow cytometry was also used to identify prostate cells in the semen of cancer patients; these studies demonstrated an ability to detect prostate cancer by utilizing differences in the PSMA/cytokeratin ratio (61). Hamdy *et al.* (62) used a monoclonal anti-PSA-antibody to sort cells according to their immunofluorescence and light-scattering properties. To establish the ploidy status, they analysed the cellular deoxyribonucleic acid content of each specimen. They found 83% of patients to be positive for PSA expressing cells and showed a higher degree of sensitivity and specificity in predicting positive bone scans than measurement of the serum PSA levels. However, they questioned the specificity of flow cytometry using anti-PSA antibodies when they compared the results of cellular analysis (75% PSA positive) with RT-PCR results (8.3% PSA positive) (63). As an explanation for the high PSA positive cell population, they suspected that PSA positive cells in the blood could represent monocytes that express PSA, either following binding of free serum PSA or phagocytosis of tumour cells. Similar results were obtained by Brandt *et al.* (64) and led this group to the development of a cytokeratin immunomagnetic bead method to isolate PSA-positive cells from the peripheral blood of prostate cancer patients. De la Taille *et al.* likewise showed that RT-PCR is superior to flow cytometry by having a detection limit of 1 LNCaP cell per 10 million lymphocytes, whereas the limit of detection for flow cytometry in their study was 1 LNCaP cell in 1,000 lymphocytes (65, 66). Racila *et al.* (67) reported a highly significant difference in the number of disseminated cells between normals and cancer (breast and prostate) patients combining immunomagnetic enrichment with multiparameter flow cytometry. In their study, disseminated epithelial cells were defined as nucleic $acid^+$, $CD45^-$ and $cytokeratin^+$. A recent study by Moreno *et al.*, using multiparameter flow cytometry demonstrated stable diurnal levels of circulating tumour cells in 8 prostate cancer patients (68). They showed a moderately good correlation between the serum PSA level and the number of disseminated tumour cells.

In summary, despite the analytical power of flow cytometry, there remain difficulties in the consistent and reproducible detection of disseminated cells (69). New technological advances are constantly being made in the hardware and software but the biggest hurdle appears to be biological; that is, identification of a marker that is highly and specifically expressed on the tumour cells of interest and one that allows viable disseminated tumour cells to be detected and sorted for further study.

Reverse Transcriptase Polymerase Chain Reaction (RT-PCR)

In recent years, RT-PCR supplanted immunohistology and flow cytometry and became the most common technique for detecting disseminated prostate cancer cells in the blood, lymph node and bone marrow (4, 31, 36, 70–73). With the first reports appearing in 1992 (30, 33), numerous studies have since demonstrated a high sensitivity and specificity for the use of RT-PCR in the detection of circulating prostate cancer cells and many suggested that haematogenous metastases may be a relatively early event in the natural history of human prostate cancer. Many studies used the messenger ribonucleic acid (mRNA) of PSA as a target of their reverse transcription to generate copy deoxyribonucleic acid (cDNA) that was amplified by the polymerase chain reaction (PCR). PSA was used because it is known to be highly expressed and nearly specific to prostate epithelial cells (27). PSA mRNA has been detected in some studies at very low abundance in non-prostatic normal and malignant tissues, including breast, lung, ovary and endometrium (27, 74–76). Although the PSA transcript is the most frequent target for prostate cancer RT-PCR studies, PSMA and human glandular kallikrein (hK2) have also been used. PSMA, a type II integral membrane protein, is expressed far more in prostatic than in other tissues, such as small intestine, brain and salivary gland (77). Human glandular kallikrein is a member of the kallikrein family of serine proteases; it shares about 80% of its DNA sequence with PSA. RT-PCR assays that target hK2 or PSA require primers that can distinguish between these similar transcripts. An excellent overview of RT-PCR for detection of circulating prostate cancer cells including primer selection, control genes, primer sequences and a discussion on the limit of detection for PSA, PSMA and hK2 was prepared by Corey and Corey in 1998 (27). As noted in this review, it is important to design appropriate controls for clinically based RT-PCR. For example, one should consider endogenous versus exogenous and internal versus external controls. An endogenous control entails the amplification of a gene that is normally present in the sample under investigation, whereas an exogenous control uses either a synthetic gene or a gene from another source that is added to the reaction. An internal control is performed in the same reaction, whereas an external control is performed separately.

Comparison of the three prostate cancer-associated markers shows the message for hK2 to be the least sensitive for the detection of circulating prostate cells (26, 78). Nevertheless, hK2 RT-PCR showed positive results in a few patients with prostate cancer, whereas PSA RT-PCR was negative in the same patients (26). Studies using PSMA as the target have been variable and somewhat controversial since the use of inappropriately selected primers, especially in early studies, resulted in a high rate of detection in normal blood cells. However, a number of PSMA studies have been published and, in general, there appears to be an increase in detection of disseminated cells among patients with advanced disease (25, 79–85). In comparing PSA RT-PCR to PSMA RT-PCR, some studies showed a higher rate of positive findings in peripheral blood samples using the PSMA RT-PCR (80–82) but other studies demonstrated that PSA is the better target and achieved a higher sensitivity (25, 83). In a recent report by Millon *et al.* (34), PSMA RT-PCR could not be used as a prognostic tool since high PSMA mRNA illegitimate expression was shown in some healthy donors. The results of representative studies using PSMA RT-PCR are shown in Table 1.

Table 1. Detection of circulating prostate cancer cells by using PSMA RT-PCR

		RT-PCR Result, Positive/Total (%)		
Reference	Sample	Localized CaP	Advanced CaP	Control
Israeli *et al.* (80)	PB	13/18 (72%)	32/57 (67%)	2/39
Cama *et al.* (25)	PB	19/80 (24%)	28/71 (39%)	0/65
Loric *et al.* (82)	PB	12/27 (44%)	28/33 (85%)	0/53
Sokoloff *et al.* (83)	PB	12/69 (17%)	13/39 (39%)	2/19
Su *et al.* (35)	PB	8/21 (38%)	not reported	not reported
Zhang *et al.* (84)	PB	11/48 (23%)	10/11 (91%)	0/20
Millon *et al.* (34)	PB	45/55 (81%), overall		14/19

Notes: PSMA, prostate specific membrane antigen; PB, peripheral blood; RT-PCR, reverse transcriptase polymerase chain reaction; CaP, prostate cancer.

Zhang *et al.* (84) reported better clinical utility by combining PSMA and PSA RT-PCR. However, most of the efforts to detect circulating prostate cancer cells in blood, bone marrow and lymph node samples of prostate cancer patients have used PSA RT-PCR (Table 2). There is still no agreement among investigators on whether PSA RT-PCR correlates with clinical stage. The issue is likely to remain unresolved since there are important differences in technique and patient selection among investigators.

Following the initial efforts to correlate RT-PCR findings with clinical stage, considerable attention was focused on determining whether RT-PCR findings obtained preoperatively correlated to clinical outcome. Olsson *et al.* (95, 96) revealed that their preoperative RT-PCR results were independent predictors of a potential postoperative treatment failure when using serum PSA levels greater than 0.2 ng/ml as an indicator of tumour recurrence; follow-up periods were 13.6 and 25.4 months, respectively. Wood *et al.* (72) also reported a significant correlation between RT-PCR results using bone marrow samples, pathological stage and serum PSA levels, finding that negative RT-PCR status was a significant predictor of disease-free survival ($p = 0.004$). The follow-up was 15.4 months. With a follow-up of 11.9 months, Katz *et al.* (73) reported the PSA RT-PCR status to be a significant predictor of surgical pathology and postoperative biochemical recurrence ($p = 0.006$). They reported a higher significance with a follow-up of 25 months (97). Okegawa and colleagues (98), using PSA and PSMA RT-PCR in peripheral blood and lymph nodes, reported a biochemical recurrence rate of 82% in patients with RT-PCR positive lymph nodes and found RT-PCR results in blood and lymph nodes to be an independent prognostic factor for biochemical recurrence. Kantoff *et al.* (99) evaluated the prognostic significance of RT-PCR for PSA mRNA in the peripheral blood of men with hormone refractory prostate cancer, and showed a significant difference in survival time: 18 months in patients who were RT-PCR negative compared to 13 months in patients who were RT-PCR positive ($p = 0.004$). Ghossein *et al.* (100) obtained similar results in

Table 2. Detection of circulating prostate cancer cells by using PSA RT-PCR

Reference	Sample	RT-PCR Result, Positive/Total (%)		Control
		Localized CaP	Advanced CaP	
Moreno *et al.* (30)	PB	not reported	4/12 (33%)	0/17
Israeli *et al.* (80)	PB	0/18 (0%)	13/46 (28%)	1/39
Katz *et al.* (86)	PB	25/65 (39%)	50/67 (75%)	0/40
Cama *et al.* (25)	PB	27/80 (34%)	54/71 (76%)	0/65
Seiden *et al.* (87)	PB	6/100 (6%)	11/35 (31%)	0/14
Ghossein *et al.* (88)	PB	6/25 (24%)	28/82 (34%)	0/27
Loric *et al.* (82)	PB	3/27 (11%)	17/33 (51%)	0/53
Olsson *et al.* (71)	PB	44/138 (32%)	100/142 (70%)	not reported
Sokoloff *et al.* (83)	PB	43/69 (62%)	29/33 (88%)	1/19
Corey *et al.* (26)	PB	12/63 (19%)	6/13 (46%)	0/20
	BM	45/63 (71%)	11/14 (79%)	0/16
Henke *et al.* (89)	PB	5/12 (42%), overall		12/31
Melchior *et al.* (29)	PB	14/71 (20%)	9/14 (64%)	0/30
	BM	44/71 (62%)	13/15 (87%)	0/30
Zhang *et al.* (84)	PB	6/48 (13%)	7/11 (64%)	0/20
Millon *et al.* (34)	PB	4/31 (13%)	5/11 (45%)	1/19
Ellis *et al.* (36)	PB	26/131 (20%)	42/115 (42%)	not reported
Wood *et al.* (90)	BM	19/43 (44%)	24/34 (71%)	0/5
Grasso *et al.* (91)	PB	37/67 (55%)	11/11 (100%)	0/35
Mejean *et al.* (92)	PB	33/99 (33%), overall		2/92
Gelmini *et al.* (93)	PB	14/44 (32%)	not reported	0/30[a]
Straub *et al.* (94)	PB	19/40 (40%)	28/40 (72%)	0/27[a]

Notes: PSA, prostate specific antigen; PB, peripheral blood; BM, bone marrow; RT-PCR, reverse transcriptase polymerase chain reaction; CaP, prostate cancer.
[a] Using real-time RT-PCR.

patients with metastatic androgen independent prostate cancer. However, many other investigators, including ourselves, conducted studies in large numbers of patients and did not find preoperative RT-PCR results to be an important prognostic factor (36, 97, 101–103). Thus, today this test cannot be recommended for routine clinical use.

Recently, there has been an increased effort to find new markers associated with prostate cancer and to utilize these in RT-PCR for detection of disseminated cells. One of these is prostasin, a 40-kD glycoprotein identified as a serine protease and purified from human semen (104). It is synthesized in prostate epithelial cells and secreted into the ducts. After full-length encoding, both the cDNA and genomic DNA have been cloned allowing the design of specific oligonucleotides for RT-PCR (105–107). Laribi *et al.* (104), using prostasin RT-PCR, demonstrated a 26% detection rate in peripheral blood for patients with localized prostate cancer and a 63% detection rate in patients with metastatic disease. All controls were negative.

Despite the encouraging data shown by some groups, there are still limitations encountered when using RT-PCR for the detection of disseminated cancer cells. Some are technical and others are biological. For example, one of the most important technical issues has been mispriming. It is especially harmful in the early amplification cycles, because the misprimed species generated will be present throughout the reaction and are likely to be amplified in some form along with the target cDNA. Mispriming both increases the noise and reduces the signal associated with the amplification of the true target. Two technical improvements that address this problem are the use of hot-start conditions and the use of nested primers.

Another technical issue relates to message abundance. While PSA and PSMA are highly expressed, other prostate cancer associated messages are in relatively low abundance, e.g., hK2. To detect low abundant messages, the RT-PCR assay must be highly optimized with primers selected with considerable care. Even after considerable effort, detection of a few cancer cells among several million-fold or more of normal peripheral blood or bone marrow cells can be a difficult task. Immunohistology and flow cytometry have a potential advantage over RT-PCR, in that they provide a quantitative assessment of the number of disseminated cells in the specimen, whereas standard RT-PCR is qualitative but more sensitive. Several recent studies have applied semi-quantitative RT-PCR to the detection of disseminated cells (93, 94, 108–111) but it is too early to determine whether this approach will add significant clinical utility. Since RT-PCR utilizes expressed transcripts as the target, it is still unknown whether an increased signal indicates a higher expression of transcript in a few cells or more cells expressing the targeted transcript.

METHODS OF CELL ENRICHMENT/ISOLATION

The discussion so far has focused on the detection of disseminated cancer cells and the correlation of their presence to clinical staging and/or risk of recurrence. While controversy remains over their clinical value, there is no doubt that these investigations have established the presence of PSA+ and PSMA+ cells in the blood and bone marrow of prostate cancer patients early in the course of the disease. Additionally, there is general agreement that men without prostate cancer do not have these circulating cells, and the proportion of prostate cancer patients who have these disseminated cells increases with stage progression and that the number of detected cells usually increases as well. Many, including ourselves, do not believe much more can be contributed to the field by the simple detection of these circulating PSA+ and/or PSMA+ cells. Despite the dozens of studies performed to date, one can still argue that there isn't conclusive proof that these disseminated cells are, in fact, prostate cancer cells and not prostate epithelial cells. The emphasis must now focus on the characterization of these disseminated cells, so that the widely held belief that epithelial cells detected in the peripheral circulation or bone marrow are indeed cancer cells will be proven correct (85, 112–115). This necessitates at the minimum, enrichment and ideally isolation of homogeneous populations and/or individual cells.

Density Gradient (non-immunological)

We previously discussed the use of density gradient centrifugation as the initial step in separating the MNC and disseminated epithelial cells from the red blood cells and granulocytes. This, of itself, is not considered enrichment. However, there have been efforts to utilize the principle of density gradient centrifugation to obtain a semi-enriched tumour cell population. For example, a commercial product similar to Ficoll-Hypaque, OncoQuick (Greiner Bio-One, Germany), was developed to achieve an enriched disseminated tumour cell population from peripheral blood. In at least one preliminary study, the purity of cells in the interphase was higher with OncoQuick than with Ficoll-Hypaque (116). Another non-immunological approach to obtain an enriched disseminated tumour cell population was described by Böckmann *et al.* (117). They used the divergent features of cancer cells in comparison to haematopoietic cells (e.g., greater size, different density, and formation of cell clusters), along with a filtration process to recover cells and cell aggregates greater than 20 μm.

Immunological Approaches

The most common approach being used to separate disseminated epithelial cells (presumed tumour cells) from the remaining cells in the specimen is based on the expression of cell-specific antigens and the recognition of these antigens by monoclonal or polyclonal antibodies. To distinguish between these cell types, one uses the presence of epithelial-specific antigens and/or the absence of haematopoietic antigens. The antibodies that recognize the target antigen are typically bound to small particles with features that allow separation of the particle-antibody-cell complex. Recently, the use of particles that become entrapped in a magnetic field have shown considerable potential in the removal of specific cell populations (85, 112, 118, 119). As mentioned previously, it is also possible to isolate the target cells using fluorescently labelled antibodies and sorting the cell mixture by flow cytometry (43, 67, 68).

The process of enriching and isolating the disseminated epithelial cells incorporates negative selection or positive selection, or a combination of both. In a negative selection scheme, cells other than the disseminated epithelial cells are targeted and selectively removed leaving behind an enriched population of the cells of interest. An example of this approach would be the targeting of the CD45 antigen that is expressed on leukocytes (67, 118). An antibody to CD61, an antigen expressed on megakaryocytes but not mononuclear cells, is recommended for a second round of negative selection when the specimen is derived from the bone marrow (118). For positive selection, the antibody would target an antigen associated with the disseminated epithelial tumour cells. They can be applied to single targets or as a mixture of antibodies targeting multiple antigens (120). The most frequently used antibodies for enrichment/isolation of disseminated prostate cancer cells include those reactive to (a) cytokeratins 8, 18, and 19, structures of the cytoskeleton, individually or to a common epitope of all three (67); and (b) human-epithelial antigen, a 34 kD epithelial glycoprotein (118, 121, 122), also called the epithelial cell adhesion molecule. Three antibodies commonly used to target different epitopes of the human epithelial antigen are designated HEA 125, BerEP4, and EpCAM (67, 114, 123, 124).

Sometimes the highest degree of enrichment is obtained by combining several approaches. As discussed subsequently, our experience in isolating prostate cancer cells from bone marrow aspirates is that negative and positive selection steps following the standard density gradient centrifugation provide a highly enriched disseminated cell population. Lansdorp *et al.* (120) noted a 1,000-fold enrichment of circulating epithelial cells from the peripheral blood by using an antibody mix of anti-CD2, anti-CD16, anti-CD19, anti-CD36, anti-CD38, anti-CD45, and anti-CD66. With this method, rosettes were formed by tetrameric antibody complexes of normal haematopoietic cells and red blood cells. Centrifugation over a Ficoll gradient resulted in an interphase containing an enriched fraction of tumour and mononuclear cells.

One should note that the literature does not use standard nomenclature when discussing enriched and isolated disseminated tumour cells. For the sake of clarity, we utilize the following scheme:

bone marrow/blood → MNC → enriched cells → pure cells

Enriched disseminated epithelial/tumour cells still represent a very heterogeneous population. By definition, there is a greater proportion of the tumour cells per non-tumour cell as found in the specimen or post standard density gradient processing but the percentage of tumour cells is most often $<0.1\%$. For detection and some characterization studies, this level of enrichment may be sufficient. However, for many investigations, especially those involving the more sophisticated techniques of molecular analyses such as gene expression microarrays, this level of enrichment is not adequate. The current challenge to those in this field is to obtain a truly homogeneous population of the cells of interest and, in some situations, to isolate and analyse single cells. Not only is this a monumental challenge, but the technology being applied for analysis must also be adapted to use very few cell numbers or even single cells. These can be huge technological hurdles but ones that must be overcome to comprehensively characterize these disseminated cancer cells and the heterogeneity that is certain to exist among this population. Our experiences in addressing these challenges are herein presented.

EFFORTS TO CHARACTERIZE THE DISSEMINATED EPITHELIAL/TUMOUR CELL POPULATION IN PATIENTS WITH PROSTATE CANCER

Fluorescence *in situ* Hybridization (FISH)

Many groups have applied immunocytogenetic approaches to help characterize disseminated prostate cancer cells (43, 49, 50, 125). Müller *et al.* (50) were the first to apply fluorescence *in situ* hybridization (FISH) to characterize disseminated prostate cancer cells. Using cytokeratin staining to identify the epithelial cells, they then attempted to determine whether these cells had an amplification of HER-2/neu by using a gene-specific DNA probe. Although they were unable to detect HER-2/neu amplification in the disseminated epithelial cells derived from prostate cancer patients, they did detect HER2/neu amplifications in two out of eight patients with breast cancer. In a later report, Müller *et al.* (49) examined numeric aberrations of chromosome 1, 7, and 8 in the bone marrow of 30 prostate cancer patients where cytokeratin positive cells were present. They reported that about 70% to 75% of cytokeratin positive cells contained chromosome 7 and 8 aneusomies. Gains of chromosome 1 occurred in 42% of these cells. Wang *et al.* (43) determined the number of androgen receptor gene copies for circulating prostate cancer cells, and although the range was from 1 to 6 copies, most of the circulating cells from the 187 patients in this series had two copies.

Reverse Transcriptase Polymerase Chain Reaction (RT-PCR)

As discussed previously, RT-PCR has frequently been used to detect the presence of disseminated prostate cancer cells in blood, bone marrow, and lymph nodes. This has been possible using un-enriched, heterogeneous cellular populations since the primary transcripts used as targets, e.g., PSA, PSMA, and hK2, are specific for epithelial-derived cells of the prostate. However, RT-PCR can also be used to help characterize these cells using markers that are not distinct to a given population, but rather infer functional status or other characteristic. Many genes that provide insight as to the character of cells are being revealed through efforts focused on gene expression micro-arrays. Since the majority of these genes are not unique to the disseminated epithelial cell population, these RT-PCR studies must be performed on homogeneous populations of disseminated cells or isolated single cells. In our laboratory, we have routinely used single-cell RT-PCR to determine gene expression in disseminated prostate cancer cells individually isolated from an enriched cell population. Sufficient RNA can be obtained from a single cell to perform multiple analyses. Several reports attest to the feasibility of single-cell RT-PCR for a variety of applications (126–128), but the application of the technique for the characterization of disseminated tumour cells is just beginning.

Telomerase Activity

Telomerase is a ribonucleoprotein that catalyses the addition of telomeric repeats to the 3′ end of chromosome DNA which then prevents the loss of telomeric sequences at each cell division. Most somatic cells lack telomerase activity after birth, but it is still expressed in proliferating cells such as activated lymphocytes, germ cells and cancer cells. A few studies have focused on telomerase activity in enriched peripheral blood cell fractions of cancer patients. Gauthier *et al.* (113) found telomerase activity in disseminated tumour cells of patients (73%) with Stage IIIB, and IV non-small cell lung cancer, and 72% of patients with a Duke's Stage C and D colon cancer. In a more recent report, Soria *et al.* (115) using the same method to harvest epithelial cells from the peripheral blood of Stage IV breast cancer patients were able to detect telomerase activity in 21 out of 25 patients. In both studies, telomerase activity was not detectable in cells from healthy volunteers. Thus, detection of telomerase activity among disseminated cells appears to be highly suggestive that the epithelial cells are cancer cells. Studies on telomerase expression in prostate cancer disseminated cells are now under way.

Comparison of Disseminated Cells to those of the Primary Tumour

One of the major questions under study is how the disseminated cancer cells compare to those of the primary tumour. Of course, there is the high probability that the disseminated cells, as the primary tumour, are a heterogeneous population with some cells being more aggressive than others. This assumption stems from studies that have shown functional and clonal heterogeneity among prostate cancer metastases (129). At this point, there are no extensive studies reporting on the comparison of disseminated cell characteristics to those of the primary tumour. Such studies will most likely require the analysis of highly purified populations of the disseminated cells by techniques such as gene expression microarrays or comparative genomic hybridization (see next section).

Genomic Alterations, Comparative Genomic Hybridization (CGHs)

A number of nucleic acid-based techniques have been applied to the detection and characterization of circulating tumour cells (130, 131). For example, these have been applied to the detection of mutations of proto-oncogenes and tumour suppressor genes (132–134) and changes of the methylation status (135). The techniques have included restriction-length polymorphism-based enriched PCR, peptide nucleic acid (PNA)-mediated amplification of mutated sequences (136), exonuclease amplification coupled capture technique (point-EXACCT) (137), mutation ligation assays (138), and allele-specific amplification (139). In addition, characterization of the disseminated cells will certainly include a determination of loss of heterozygosity (LOH) and microsatellite instability (MIN), as these alterations have been associated with a worse prognosis (140).

Two relatively new techniques will have considerable impact on the characterization of the disseminated cancer cells. One that we have previously mentioned is cDNA array hybridization, often referred to as gene expression micro-arrays. Using 'gene chips', this technique allows one to assess gene expression levels of several thousand genes in a single assay. Many investigators are utilizing this technique for the analysis of gene expression in human tumours. Recent studies indicate that this approach is robust and highly reproducible as demonstrated by recent reports evaluating a subset of androgen-regulated genes with prostate-enhanced expression such as TMPRSS2 (141), PART-1 (142), and PSDR1 (143). At the present time, the analysis of disseminated cells by gene expression micro-arrays is a technical challenge due to the necessity of having a homogeneous population of cells and a large number of cells from which to extract sufficient RNA for evaluation. However, a wealth of information awaits those who can meet this challenge.

The second major advance is in the field of comparative genomic hybridization (CGH), where array CGH has shown tremendous potential for detecting chromosomal alterations. Array CGH cannot be easily applied to direct studies of disseminated cells due to many of the same technical limitations confronting gene expression micro-arrays. However, rapid advances are being made in this area. For example, Klein *et al.* (144) adapted CGH for single isolated cells from cancer patients and detected more chromosomal aberrations than when they used a pool of tumour cells. Also, Hodgson *et al.* (145) have recently demonstrated the feasibility of correctly detecting copy-number status using array CGH when the percentage of tumour cell DNA was as low as 40% of the total DNA in the sample. This is a significant finding since it alleviates somewhat the need for a homogeneous population of cells for such studies. There is great anticipation that these techniques will provide considerable new information on the characterization of circulating tumour cells in the near future. Our group is actively exploring array CGH for the study of disseminated prostate cancer cells.

Single-cell Isolation – the Seattle Experience

The procedure we are currently using at the University of Washington in Seattle, USA for the characterization of disseminated prostate cancer cells is a combination of several approaches described in the preceding text and illustrated in Figure 1. The initial steps are slightly different depending upon whether the specimen is peripheral blood or a bone marrow aspirate, and these are described separately in the following two paragraphs.

Peripheral blood is collected in a vacutainer cell preparation tube (CPT) containing 0.1 M sodium citrate anticoagulant and a blood separation media composed

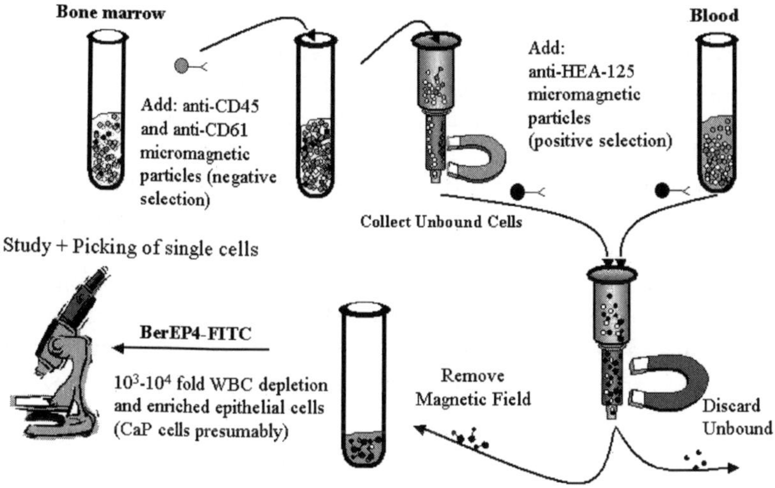

Figure 1. Algorithm to enrich and isolate circulating tumour cells from the peripheral blood and bone marrow of prostate cancer patients presently used at the University of Washington, Seattle, USA.

of a thixotropicpolyester gel and Ficoll-Hypaque solution (Becton Dickinson, #362761). The tubes are centrifuged for 30 minutes at 1,800 g. The mononuclear cells and disseminated tumour cells are taken off and washed. Anti-Human epithelial antigen (anti-HEA) antibody coated paramagnetic microbeads (MACS, Miltenyi Biotec, Germany), along with a FcR-blocking reagent, are added to the cells and incubated for 30 minutes.

A bone marrow aspirate is obtained from one or both iliac crests. The bone marrow is collected in a syringe which contains 10 ml of 6% sodium citrate. The contents are transferred to a 50 cc tube, underlayed with 15 ml of Ficoll-Hypaque and centrifuged at 400 g for 30 minutes. The interphase layer consisting of MNC and circulating tumour cells is recovered and washed. Paramagnetic microparticles labelled with anti-CD45 and anti-CD61 antibodies, reactive with common leukocytes and megakaryocytes respectively, are added to the cells as an initial negative selection process. The cell preparation is passed through a magnetic field column (MACS, Miltenyi Biotec, Germany); the CD45 and CD61 positive cells are retained, whereas the disseminated epithelial/cancer cells pass through and are collected. In preparation for positive selection, anti-HEA antibody coated microparticles and the FcR-blocking reagent are mixed with these cells. From this point forward, the processing of the bone marrow and blood samples is the same.

Positive selection involves passing the anti-HEA microparticle cell mixture over a magnetic field column. Epithelial/tumour cells are retained, while non-HEA expressing cells flow through. Collection of the HEA positive cells occurs when the magnetic field is removed and the column is rinsed. We have used the prostate cancer cell line LNCaP to test these methods. Upon spiking

LNCaP cells into normal bone marrow or peripheral blood specimens, we can consistently achieve at least a 10^3 to 10^4-fold enriched tumour cell fraction with approximately an 80% to 90% recovery of the LNCaP cells.

The enriched cell population is divided into three equal parts: one is used for PSA RT-PCR, the second is further processed with cytospin and used for immunohistochemistry (e.g., anti-PSA; see Figure 2) and the third is used for the isolation of single disseminated epithelial cells. This is accomplished by adding FITC labelled anti-BerEP4 antibodies to the cells. The cells are kept on ice and viewed under fluorescent light using an inverted microscope equipped with a micromanipulator pipette system. The BerEP4 positive epithelial/tumour cells are detected (Figure 3a,b) and counted. Using the pipette system individual cells are picked (Figure 4) and combined for pooled cell studies or analysed as single cells.

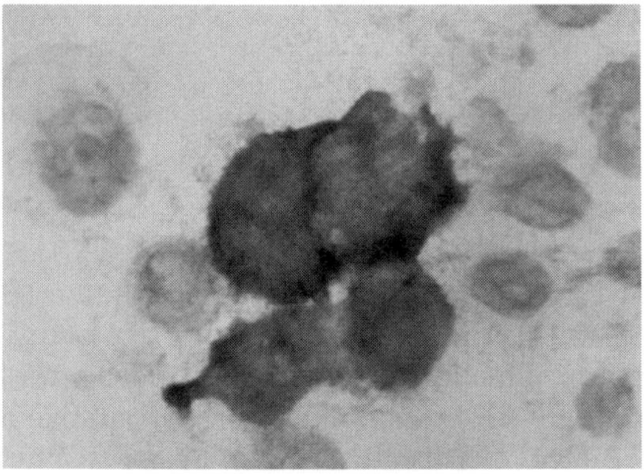

Figure 2. Immunohistochemistry showing PSA positive cell cluster in the enriched cell population from the peripheral blood of a patient with prostate cancer, ×40.

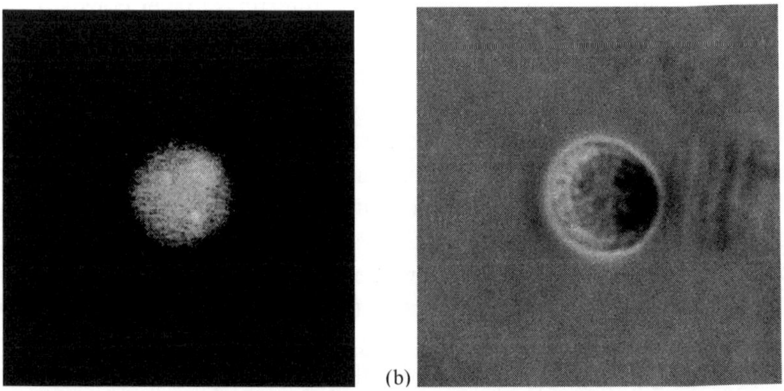

(a) (b)

Figure 3a,b. The same epithelial cell from the bone marrow of a prostate cancer patient BerEP4-FITC labelled (a) and with phase contrast microscopy (b), ×40.

Using the method described above, we evaluated a series of peripheral blood specimens from 138 patients and bone marrow aspirates from 126 patients (118). The great majority of these were from patients with prostate cancer but we also included as controls patients with other cancers, patients with benign prostatic hyperplasia, and normal subjects. We found that 83% of the pre-radical prostatectomy patients were positive for epithelial/tumour cells in their bone marrow samples and 51% in their blood samples. However, approximately 20% of the bone marrow specimens yielded epithelial staining that was very weak and upon further analysis these cells may be judged as background staining. This compared to PSA RT-PCR positivity rates using an aliquot of the non-enriched cell population from these patients of 64% in bone marrow and 44% in blood. Most of the patients that scored positive for disseminated epithelial cells were also positive by PSA immunohistochemistry: 77% in the bone marrow, and 87% in the blood. We have been intrigued to find BerEP4 positive cells in bone marrow (87%) and blood samples (20%) more than five years after radical prostatectomy in patients without any clinical signs of recurrent disease. Epithelial/tumour cells were detected in all patients who had advanced metastatic prostate cancer. PSA RT-PCR showed positive results in 93% of these patients. Overall, the number of disseminated cells detected in the specimens vary widely. In the pre-surgery patients the range is several dozen to several hundred in the bone marrow specimens and approximately 10% to 20% of this yield in peripheral blood. The advanced disease patients can yield into the thousands of BerEP4 positive cells in the bone marrow specimens. In contrast, during follow-up where there is no clinical indication of disease, fewer than a dozen cells are usually detected in the bone marrow aspirates. Throughout this total series, control specimens (i.e., from patients with other cancers, BPH, and healthy subjects) were negative for PSA-RT-PCR in all cases. Only one epithelial cell was detected in

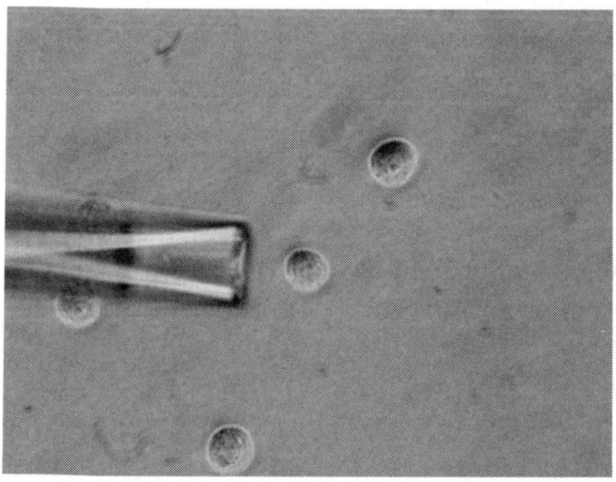

Figure 4. Micropipette-tip (orifice 30 μm) picking a single prostate cancer cell (LNCaP) for further examination, × 40.

the blood of 52 healthy donors, but it was not PSA positive. Among 16 control bone marrow aspirates, only one had evidence of epithelial cell presence, and in that specimen only 2 epithelial cells were detected. Neither was PSA positive.

Our data show epithelial cells of presumably prostate cancer origin are commonly detected in the blood and bone marrow of men prior to radical prostatectomy and in a large percentage of patients many years following surgery. However, it is clear that not all of these cells will contribute to the development of metastases, as the percentage of patients with cells detected prior to radical prostatectomy is higher than the expected failure rate. It is conceivable that some of these cells will become dormant and persist for many years without disease progression or metastases. We have further demonstrated a procedure where one can effectively isolate single disseminated cells to analyse individually or to pool together. The aim of future studies in our group is to differentiate between the disseminated cells that are most likely to lead to metastases from those that are indolent.

CONCLUSION

The data from many laboratories consistently demonstrate the presence of disseminated epithelial/tumour cells in patients with prostate cancer very early in their disease course. The bone marrow appears to be a richer source of these disseminated cells than the peripheral blood and detection of these cells is possible even years after radical prostatectomy in patients who have no signs of clinical disease. Although studies such as RT-PCR demonstrate the presence of these cells in many, if not most, pre-surgical patients, only a few studies have shown a correlation between the presence of these cells and stage or risk of progression. However, many questions have arisen concerning the character of these disseminated cells and much effort is now being expended to define their properties. These are not easy tasks since many of the techniques require homogeneous cell populations and hundreds, if not thousands, of cells. Towards this end, investigators are attempting to isolate disseminated cells using a variety of enrichment techniques and others are developing the technology for characterizing pools of a few dozen cells and even single cells. Without question, techniques such as gene expression micro-arrays and array CGH, once adapted for the study of disseminated cells, will add considerable and valuable information on topics including virulence, progression to androgen independence, trafficking, cellular heterogeneity and dormancy. From these forthcoming studies one may be able to: (1) determine prognostic information, (2) provide new information on the biology of metastases, and (3) provide insights leading to novel therapeutic opportunities. Due to the relatively slow-growing nature of micrometastatic prostate cancer, the presence of PSA as a serum marker and the proclivity of metastases to go to bone, the further study of disseminated tumour cells and application of the acquired knowledge appears ideally suited for this patient group.

REFERENCES

1. Greenlee RT, Hill-Harmon MB, Murray T, Thun M. Cancer statistics, 2001. CA Cancer J Clin. 2001; 51: 15–36.
2. Smith RA, von Eschenbach AC, Wender R, Levin B, Byers T, Rothenberger D, Brooks, D, Creasman W, Cohen C, Runowicz C, Saslow D, Cokkinides V, Eyre H. American Cancer Society guidelines for the early detection of cancer: update of early detection guidelines for prostate, colorectal, and endometrial cancers. Also: update. 2001 – testing for early lung cancer detection. CA Cancer J Clin. 2001; 51: 38–75.
3. Parker SL, Tong T, Bolden S, Wingo PA. Cancer statistics, 1997. CA Cancer J Clin. 1997; 47: 5–27.
4. Raj GV, Moreno JG, Gomella LG. Utilization of polymerase chain reaction technology in the detection of solid tumors. Cancer. 1998; 82: 1419–1442.
5. Pienta KJ. Etiology, epidemiology, and prevention of carcinoma of the prostate. In: Walsh PC, Retik AB, Vaughan ED, Wein AJ, editors. Campbell's Urology. New York: Saunders; 1997, pp. 2489–2496.
6. Han M, Partin AW, Pound CR, Epstein JI, Walsh PC. Long-term biochemical disease-free and cancer-specific survival following anatomic radical retropubic prostatectomy. The 15-year Johns Hopkins experience. Urol Clin North Am. 2001; 28:555–565.
7. Lepor H. Radical retropubic prostatectomy. Urol Clin North Am. 2001; 28: 509–519, viii.
8. Walsh PC, Marschke P, Ricker D, Burnett AL. Patient-reported urinary continence and sexual function after anatomic radical prostatectomy. Urology. 2000; 55: 58–61.
9. Gallucci M, Vincenzoni A. Laparoscopic radical prostatectomy: a marketing or surgical strategy? Curr Opin Urol. 2001; 11: 305–308.
10. Olsson LE, Salomon L, Nadu A, Hoznek A, Cicco A, Saint F, Chopin D, Abbou CC. Prospective patient-reported continence after laparoscopic radical prostatectomy. Urology. 2001; 58: 570–572.
11. Turk I, Deger S, Winkelmann B, Schonberger B, Loening SA. Laparoscopic Radical Prostatectomy. Technical aspects and experience with 125 cases. Eur Urol. 2001; 40: 46–53.
12. Turk I, Deger IS, Winkelmann B, Roigas J, Schonberger B, Loening SA. [Laparoscopic radical prostatectomy. Experiences with 145 interventions]. Urologe A. 2001; 40: 199–206.
13. Lee WR, Hall MC, McQuellon RP, Case LD, McCullough DL. A prospective quality-of-life study in men with clinically localized prostate carcinoma treated with radical prostatectomy, external beam radiotherapy, or interstitial brachytherapy. Int J Radiat Oncol Biol Phys. 2001; 51: 614–623.
14. Siegsmund M, Musial A, Weiss J, Alken P. [Ldr brachytherapy, a minimally invasive alternative in the treatment of organ-confined prostate cancer]. Onkologie. 2001; 24 Suppl 5: 46–50.
15. Dejter SW, Jr, Cunningham RE, Noguchi PD, Jones RV, Moul JW, McLeod DG, Lynch JH. Prognostic significance of DNA ploidy in carcinoma of prostate. Urology. 1989; 33: 361–366.
16. Kasahara K, Taguchi T, Yamasaki I, Karashima T, Kamada M, Yuri K, Shuin T. Fluorescence in situ hybridization to assess transitional changes of aneuploidy for chromosomes 7, 8, 10, 12, 16, X and Y in metastatic prostate cancer following antiandrogen therapy. Int J Oncol. 2001; 19: 543–549.

17. Alcaraz A, Takahashi S, Brown JA, Herath JF, Bergstralh EJ, Larson-Keller JJ, Lieber MM, Jenkins RB. Aneuploidy and aneusomy of chromosome 7 detected by fluorescence in situ hybridization are markers of poor prognosis in prostate cancer. Cancer Res. 1994; 54: 3998–4002.
18. Takahashi S, Alcaraz A, Brown JA, Borell TJ, Herath JF, Bergstralh EJ, Lieber MM, Jenkins RB. Aneusomies of chromosomes 8 and Y detected by fluorescence in situ hybridization are prognostic markers for pathological stage C (pt3N0M0) prostate carcinoma. Clin Cancer Res. 1996; 2: 137–145.
19. Lerner SE, Blute ML, Bergstralh EJ, Bostwick DG, Eickholt JT, Zincke H. Analysis of risk factors for progression in patients with pathologically confined prostate cancers after radical retropubic prostatectomy. J Urol. 1996; 156: 137–143.
20. Bretton PR, Melamed MR, Fair WR, Cote RJ. Detection of occult micrometastases in the bone marrow of patients with prostate carcinoma. Prostate. 1994; 25: 108–114.
21. Kollermann J, Heseding B, Helpap B, Kollermann MW, Pantel K. Comparative immunocytochemical assessment of isolated carcinoma cells in lymph nodes and bone marrow of patients with clinically localized prostate cancer. Int J Cancer. 1999; 84: 145–149.
22. Pantel K, Aignherr C, Kollermann J, Caprano J, Riethmuller G, Kollermann MW. Immunocytochemical detection of isolated tumour cells in bone marrow of patients with untreated stage C prostatic cancer. Eur J Cancer. 1995; 31A: 1627–1632.
23. Pantel K, Izbicki J, Passlick B, Angstwurm M, Haussinger K, Thetter O, Riethmuller G. Frequency and prognostic significance of isolated tumour cells in bone marrow of patients with non-small-cell lung cancer without overt metastases. Lancet. 1996; 347: 649–653.
24. Pantel K, Enzmann T, Kollermann J, Caprano J, Riethmuller G, Kollermann MW. Immunocytochemical monitoring of micrometastatic disease: reduction of prostate cancer cells in bone marrow by androgen deprivation. Int J Cancer. 1997; 71: 521–525.
25. Cama C, Olsson CA, Raffo AJ, Perlman H, Buttyan R, O'Toole K, McMahon D, Benson MC, Katz, AE. Molecular staging of prostate cancer. II. A comparison of the application of an enhanced reverse transcriptase polymerase chain reaction assay for prostate specific antigen versus prostate specific membrane antigen. J Urol. 1995; 153: 1373–1378.
26. Corey E, Arfman EW, Oswin MM, Melchior SW, Tindall DJ, Young CY, Ellis WJ, Vessella RL. Detection of circulating prostate cells by reverse transcriptase-polymerase chain reaction of human glandular kallikrein (hK2) and prostate-specific antigen (PSA) messages. Urology. 1997; 50: 184–188.
27. Corey E, Corey MJ. Detection of disseminated prostate cells by reverse transcription-polymerase chain reaction (RT-PCR): technical and clinical aspects. Int J Cancer. 1998; 77: 655–673.
28. Ghossein RA, Carusone L, Bhattacharya S. Molecular detection of micrometastases and circulating tumor cells in melanoma prostatic and breast carcinomas. In Vivo. 2000; 14: 237–250.
29. Melchior SW, Corey E, Ellis WJ, Ross AA, Layton TJ, Oswin MM, Lange PH, Vessella RL. Early tumor cell dissemination in patients with clinically localized carcinoma of the prostate. Clin Cancer Res. 1997; 3: 249–256.
30. Moreno JG, Croce CM, Fischer R, Monne M, Vihko P, Mulholland SG, Gomella LG. Detection of hematogenous micrometastasis in patients with prostate cancer. Cancer Res. 1992; 52: 6110–6112.

31. Oefelein MG, Kaul K, Herz B, Blum MD, Holland JM, Keeler TC, Cook WA, Ignatoff JM. Molecular detection of prostate epithelial cells from the surgical field and peripheral circulation during radical prostatectomy. J Urol. 1996; 155: 238–242.
32. Olsson CA, de Vries GM, Raffo AJ, Benson MC, O'Toole K, Cao Y, Buttyan RE, Katy AE. Preoperative reverse transcriptase polymerase chain reaction for prostate specific antigen predicts treatment failure following radical prostatectomy. J Urol. 1996; 155: 1557–1562.
33. Vessella RL, Riley DE, Blouke KA, Arfman EW, Lange PH. A sensitive method for detection of a prostate tumor cell marker using the polymerase chain reaction. J Urol. 1992; 147 suppl.: 441A.
34. Millon R, Jacqmin D, Muller D, Guillot J, Eber M, Abecassis J. Detection of prostate-specific antigen-or prostate-specific membrane antigen-positive circulating cells in prostatic cancer patients: clinical implications. Eur Urol. 1999; 36: 278–285.
35. Su SL, Heston WD, Perrotti M, Cookson MS, Stroumbakis N, Huyrk R, Edwards E, Brander B, Coke J, Soloway S, Lewis A, Fair WR, Perroti M. Evaluating neoadjuvant therapy effectiveness on systemic disease: use of a prostatic-specific membrane reverse transcription polymerase chain reaction. Urology. 1997; 49: 95–101.
36. Ellis WJ, Vessella RL, Corey E, Arfman EW, Oswin MM, Melchior S, Lange PH. The value of a reverse transcriptase polymerase chain reaction assay in preoperative staging and followup of patients with prostate cancer. J Urol. 1998; 159: 1134–1138.
37. Bianco FJ, Jr, Wood DP, Jr, Gomes DO, Nemeth JA, Beaman AA, Cher ML. Proliferation of prostate cancer cells in the bone marrow predicts recurrence in patients with localized prostate cancer. Prostate. 2001; 49: 235–242.
38. Belldegrun A, Bander NH, Lerner SP, Wood DP, Pantuck AJ. Society of Urologic Oncology Biotechnology Forum: new approaches and targets for advanced prostate cancer. J Urol. 2001; 166: 1316–1321.
39. Gong MC, Chang SS, Watt F, O'Keefe DS, Bacich DJ, Uchida A, Bander NH, Reuter VE, Gaudin PB, Molloy PL, Sadelian M, Heston WD. Overview of evolving strategies incorporating prostate-specific membrane antigen as target for therapy. Mol Urol. 2000; 4: 217–222.
40. Boyum A. Isolation of lymphocytes, granulocytes and macrophages. Scand J Immunol. 1976; Suppl. 5: 9–15.
41. Boyum A, Lovhaug D, Tresland L, Nordlic EM. Separation of leucocytes: improved cell purity by fine adjustments of gradient medium density and osmolality. Scand J Immunol. 1991; 34: 697–712.
42. Berteau P, Dumas F, Gala JL, Eschwege P, Lacour B, Philippe M, Loric S. Molecular detection of circulating prostate cells in cancer II: Comparison of prostate epithelial cells isolation procedures. Clin Chem. 1998; 44: 1750–1753.
43. Wang ZP, Eisenberger MA, Carducci MA, Partin AW, Scher HI, Ts'o PO. Identification and characterization of circulating prostate carcinoma cells. Cancer. 2000; 88: 2787–2795.
44. Molino A, Colombatti M, Bonetti F, Zardini M, Pasini F, Perini A, Pelosi G, Tridente G, Veneri D, Cetto GL. A comparative analysis of three different techniques for the detection of breast cancer cells in bone marrow. Cancer. 1991; 67: 1033–1036.
45. Schlimok G, Funke I, Holzmann B, Gottlinger G, Schmidt G, Hauser H, Swierkot S, Warnecke HH, Schneider B, Koprowski H. Micrometastatic cancer cells in bone marrow: in vitro detection with anti-cytokeratin and in vivo labeling with anti-17-1A monoclonal antibodies. Proc Natl Acad Sci USA. 1987; 84: 8672–8676.

46. Oberneder R, Riesenberg R, Kriegmair M, Bitzer U, Klammert R, Schneede P, Hofstetter A, Riethmuller G, Pantel K. Immunocytochemical detection and phenotypic characterization of micrometastatic tumour cells in bone marrow of patients with prostate cancer. Urol Res. 1994; 22: 3–8.
47. Pantel K, Schlimok G, Angstwurm M, Weckermann D, Schmaus W, Gath H, Passlick B, Izbicki JR, Riethmuller G. Methodological analysis of immunocytochemical screening for disseminated epithelial tumor cells in bone marrow. J Hematother. 1994; 3: 165–173.
48. Pantel K, Riethmuller G. Micrometastasis detection and treatment with monoclonal antibodies. Curr Top Microbiol Immunol. 1996; 213 (Pt 3): 1–18.
49. Müller P, Carroll P, Bowers E, Moore D, Cher M, Presti J, Wessman M, Pallavicini MG. Low frequency epithelial cells in bone marrow aspirates from prostate carcinoma patients are cytogenetically aberrant. Cancer. 1998; 83: 538–546.
50. Müller P, Weckermann D, Riethmuller G, Schlimok G. Detection of genetic alterations in micrometastatic cells in bone marrow of cancer patients by fluorescence in situ hybridization. Cancer Genet Cytogenet. 1996; 88: 8–16.
51. Murphy GP, Greene TG, Tino WT, Boynton AL, Holmes EH. Isolation and characterization of monoclonal antibodies specific for the extracellular domain of prostate specific membrane antigen. J Urol. 1998; 160: 2396–2401.
52. Pantel K, Schlimok G, Angstwurm M, Passlick B, Izbicki JR, Johnson JP, Riethmuller G. Early metastasis of human solid tumours: expression of cell adhesion molecules. Ciba Found Symp. 1995; 189: 157–170.
53. Weckermann D, Müller P, Wawroschek F, Krawczak G, Riethmuller G, Schlimok G. Micrometastases of bone marrow in localized prostate cancer: correlation with established risk factors. J Clin Oncol. 1999; 17: 3438–3443.
54. Weckermann D, Wawroschek F, Krawczak G, Haude KH, Harzmann R. Does the immunocytochemical detection of epithelial cells in bone marrow (micrometastasis) influence the time to biochemical relapse after radical prostatectomy? Urol Res. 1999; 27: 285–290.
55. Weckermann D, Müller P, Wawroschek F, Harzmann R, Riethmuller G, Schlimok G. Disseminated cytokeratin positive tumor cells in the bone marrow of patients with prostate cancer: detection and prognostic value. J Urol. 2001; 166: 699–703.
56. Fordham MV, Burdge AH, Matthews J, Williams G, Cooke T. Prostatic carcinoma cell DNA content measured by flow cytometry and its relation to clinical outcome. Brit J Surg. 1986; 73: 400–403.
57. Lee SE, Currin SM, Paulson DF, Walther PJ. Flow cytometric determination of ploidy in prostatic adenocarcinoma: a comparison with seminal vesicle involvement and histopathological grading as a predictor of clinical recurrence. J Urol. 1988; 140: 769–774.
58. Liu AY, True LD, LaTray L, Ellis WJ, Vessella RL, Lange PH, Higano CS, Hood L, van den Engh G. Analysis and sorting of prostate cancer cell types by flow cytometry. Prostate. 1999; 40: 192–199.
59. Liu AY. Differential expression of cell surface molecules in prostate cancer cells. Cancer Res. 2000; 60: 3429–3434.
60. Liu AY, Peehl DM. Characterization of cultured human prostatic epithelial cells by cluster designation antigen expression. Cell Tissue Res. 2001; 305: 389–397.
61. Barren RJ, III, Holmes EH, Boynton AL, Gregorakis A, Elgamal AA, Cobb OE, Wilson CL, Ragde H, Murphy GP. Method for identifying prostate cells in semen using flow cytometry. Prostate. 1998; 36: 181–188.

62. Hamdy FC, Lawry J, Anderson JB, Parsons MA, Rees RC, Williams JL. Circulating prostate specific antigen-positive cells correlate with metastatic prostate cancer. Brit J Urol. 1992; 69: 392–396.
63. Fadlon EJ, Rees RC, McIntyre C, Sharrard RM, Lawry J, Hamdy FC. Detection of circulating prostate-specific antigen-positive cells in patients with prostate cancer by flow cytometry and reverse transcription polymerase chain reaction. Brit J Cancer. 1996; 74: 400–405.
64. Brandt B, Junker R, Griwatz C, Heidl S, Brinkmann O, Semjonow A, Assmann G, Zanker KS. Isolation of prostate-derived single cells and cell clusters from human peripheral blood. Cancer Res. 1996; 56: 4556–4561.
65. De La Taille, Muscatelli B, Colombel M, Jouault H, Amsellem S, Mazeman E, Abbou CC, Chopin D. [In vitro detection of prostate cancer circulating cells by immunocytochemistry, flow cytometry and RT-PCR PSA]. Prog Urol. 1998; 8: 1058–1064.
66. De La Taille, Salomon L, Colombel M, Abbou CC, Chopin D, Groux-Muscatelli B. [Detection of circulating prostatic cells with RT-PCR PSA in prostatic cancer]. Prog Urol. 1999; 9: 1084–1089.
67. Racila E, Euhus D, Weiss AJ, Rao C, McConnell J, Terstappen LW, Uhr JW. Detection and characterization of carcinoma cells in the blood. Proc Natl Acad Sci USA. 1998; 95: 4589–4594.
68. Moreno JG, O'Hara SM, Gross S, Doyle G, Fritsche H, Gomella LG, Terstappen LW. Changes in circulating carcinoma cells in patients with metastatic prostate cancer correlate with disease status. Urology. 2001; 58: 386–392.
69. Kostler WJ, Brodowicz T, Hejna M, Wiltschke C, Zielinski CC. Detection of minimal residual disease in patients with cancer: a review of techniques, clinical implications, and emerging therapeutic consequences. Cancer Detect Prev. 2000; 24: 376–403.
70. Ghossein RA, Carusone L, Bhattacharya S. Review: polymerase chain reaction detection of micrometastases and circulating tumor cells: application to melanoma, prostate, and thyroid carcinomas. Diagn Mol Pathol. 1999; 8: 165–175.
71. Olsson CA, de Vries GM, Benson MC, Raffo A, Buttyan R, Cama C, O'Toole K, Katz AE. The use of RT-PCR for prostate-specific antigen assay to predict potential surgical failures before radical prostatectomy: molecular staging of prostate cancer. Brit J Urol. 1996; 77: 411–417.
72. Wood DP, Jr, Banerjee M. Presence of circulating prostate cells in the bone marrow of patients undergoing radical prostatectomy is predictive of disease-free survival. J Clin Oncol. 1997; 15: 3451–3457.
73. Katz AE, de Vries GM, Benson MC, Buttyan RE, O'Toole K, Rubin MA, Stifelman M, Olsson CA. The role of the reverse-transcriptase polymerase chain reaction assay for prostate-specific antigen in the selection of patients for radical prostatectomy. Urol Clin North Am. 1996; 23: 541–549.
74. Clements J, Mukhtar A. Glandular kallikreins and prostate-specific antigen are expressed in the human endometrium. J Clin Endocrinol Metab. 1994; 78: 1536–1539.
75. Lehrer S, Terk M, Piccoli SP, Song HK, Lavagnini P, Luderer AA. Reverse transcriptase-polymerase chain reaction for prostate-specific antigen may be a prognostic indicator in breast cancer. Brit J Cancer. 1996; 74: 871–873.
76. Levesque M, Hu H, D'Costa M, Diamandis EP. Prostate-specific antigen expression by various tumors. J Clin Lab Anal. 1995; 9: 123–128.

77. Fair WR, Israeli RS, Heston WD. Prostate-specific membrane antigen. Prostate. 1997; 32: 140–148.
78. Kawakami M, Okaneya T, Furihata K, Nishizawa O, Katsuyama T. Detection of prostate cancer cells circulating in peripheral blood by reverse transcription-PCR for hKLK2. Cancer Res. 1997; 57: 4167–4170.
79. Cama C, Olsson CA, Buttyan R, de Vries GM, Wise GJ, Katz AE. Molecular staging of prostate cancer. III. Effects of cystoscopy and needle biopsy on the enhanced reverse transcriptase polymerase chain reaction assay. J Urol. 1997; 157: 1748–1751.
80. Israeli RS, Miller WH, Jr, Su SL, Powell CT, Fair WR, Samadi DS, Huryk RF, DeBlasio A, Edwards ET, Wise GJ. Sensitive nested reverse transcription polymerase chain reaction detection of circulating prostatic tumor cells: comparison of prostate- specific membrane antigen and prostate-specific antigen-based assays. Cancer Res. 1994; 54: 6306–6310.
81. Israeli RS, Miller WH, Jr, Su SL, Samadi DS, Powell CT, Heston WD, Wise GJ, Fair WR. Sensitive detection of prostatic hematogenous tumor cell dissemination using prostate specific antigen and prostate specific membrane-derived primers in the polymerase chain reaction. J Urol. 1995; 153: 573–577.
82. Loric S, Dumas F, Eschwege P, Blanchet P, Benoit G, Jardin A, Lacour B. Enhanced detection of hematogenous circulating prostatic cells in patients with prostate adenocarcinoma by using nested reverse transcription polymerase chain reaction assay based on prostate-specific membrane antigen. Clin Chem. 1995; 41: 1698–1704.
83. Sokoloff MH, Tso CL, Kaboo R, Nelson S, Ko J, Dorey F, Figlin RA, Pang S, deKernion J, Belldegrun A. Quantitative polymerase chain reaction does not improve preoperative prostate cancer staging: a clinicopathological molecular analysis of 121 patients. J Urol. 1996; 156: 1560–1566.
84. Zhang Y, Zippe CD, Van Lente F, Klein EA, Gupta MK. Combined nested reverse transcription-PCR assay for prostate-specific antigen and prostate-specific membrane antigen in detecting circulating prostatic cells. Clin Cancer Res. 1997; 3: 1215–1220.
85. Ghossein RA, Osman I, Bhattacharya S, Ferrara J, Fazzari M, Cordon-Cardo C, Scher HI. Detection of prostatic specific membrane antigen messenger RNA using immunobead reverse transcriptase polymerase chain reaction. Diagn Mol Pathol. 1999; 8: 59–65.
86. Katz AE, Olsson CA, Raffo AJ, Cama C, Perlman H, Seaman E, O'Toole KM, McMahon D, Benson MC, Buttyan R. Molecular staging of prostate cancer with the use of an enhanced reverse transcriptase-PCR assay. Urology. 1994; 43: 765–775.
87. Seiden MV, Kantoff PW, Krithivas K, Propert K, Bryant M, Haltom E, Gaynes L, Kaplan I, Bubley G, DeWolf W. Detection of circulating tumor cells in men with localized prostate cancer. J Clin Oncol. 1994; 12: 2634–2639.
88. Ghossein RA, Scher HI, Gerald WL, Kelly WK, Curley T, Amsterdam A, Zhang ZF, Rosai J. Detection of circulating tumor cells in patients with localized and metastatic prostatic carcinoma: clinical implications. J Clin Oncol. 1995; 13: 1195–2000.
89. Henke W, Jung M, Jung K, Lein M, Schlechte H, Berndt C, Rudolph B, Schnorr D, Loening SA. Increased analytical sensitivity of RT-PCR of PSA mRNA decreases diagnostic specificity of detection of prostatic cells in blood. Int J Cancer. 1997; 70: 52–56.
90. Wood DP, Jr, Banks ER, Humphreys S, Rangnekar VM. Sensitivity of immunohistochemistry and polymerase chain reaction in detecting prostate cancer cells in bone marrow. J Histochem Cytochem. 1994; 42: 505–511.

91. Grasso YZ, Gupta MK, Levin HS, Zippe CD, Klein EA. Combined nested RT-PCR assay for prostate-specific antigen and prostate-specific membrane antigen in prostate cancer patients: correlation with pathological stage. Cancer Res. 1998; 58: 1456–1459.
92. Mejean A, Vona G, Nalpas B, Damotte D, Brousse N, Chretien Y, Dufour B, Lacour B, Brechot C, Paterlini-Brechot P. Detection of circulating prostate derived cells in patients with prostate adenocarcinoma is an independent risk factor for tumor recurrence. J Urol. 2000; 163: 2022–2029.
93. Gelmini S, Tricarico C, Vona G, Livi L, Melina AD, Serni S, Cellai E, Magrini S, Villari D, Carini M, Serio M, Forti G, Pazzagli M, Orlando C. Real-Time quantitative reverse transcriptase-polymerase chain reaction (RT-PCR) for the measurement of prostate-specific antigen mRNA in the peripheral blood of patients with prostate carcinoma using the taqman detection system. Clin Chem Lab Med. 2001; 39: 385–391.
94. Straub B, Muller M, Krause H, Schrader M, Goessl C, Heicappell R, Miller K. Detection of prostate-specific antigen RNA before and after radical retropubic prostatectomy and transurethral resection of the prostate using 'Light-Cycler'-based quantitative real-time polymerase chain reaction. Urology. 2001; 58: 815–820.
95. De La Taille, Olsson CA, Buttyan R, Benson MC, Bagiella E, Cao Y, Burchardt M, Chopin DK, Katz AE. Blood-based reverse transcriptase polymerase chain reaction assays for prostatic specific antigen: long term follow-up confirms the potential utility of this assay in identifying patients more likely to have biochemical recurrence (rising PSA) following radical prostatectomy. Int J Cancer. 1999; 84: 360–364.
96. Olsson CA, de Vries GM, Raffo AJ, Benson MC, O'Toole K, Cao Y, Buttyan RE, Katz AE. Preoperative reverse transcriptase polymerase chain reaction for prostate specific antigen predicts treatment failure following radical prostatectomy. J Urol. 1996; 155: 1557–1562.
97. De La Taille, Olsson CA, Katz AE. Molecular staging of prostate cancer: dream or reality? Oncology (Huntingt). 1999; 13: 187–194.
98. Okegawa T, Nutahara K, Higashihara E. Preoperative nested reverse transcription-polymerase chain reaction for prostate specific membrane antigen predicts biochemical recurrence after radical prostatectomy. BJU Int. 1999; 84: 112–117.
99. Kantoff PW, Halabi S, Farmer DA, Hayes DF, Vogelzang NA, Small EJ. Prognostic significance of reverse transcriptase polymerase chain reaction for prostate-specific antigen in men with hormone-refractory prostate cancer. J Clin Oncol. 2001; 19: 3025–3028.
100. Ghossein RA, Rosai J, Scher HI, Seiden M, Zhang ZF, Sun M, Chang G, Berlane K, Krithivas K, Kantoff PW. Prognostic significance of detection of prostate-specific antigen transcripts in the peripheral blood of patients with metastatic androgen-independent prostatic carcinoma. Urology. 1997; 50: 100–105.
101. Hedican SP, Nelson JB, Marshke P, Carter HB, Walsh PC, Partin AW, Luo G, Veltri RW, O'Hara SM. Evaluation of preoperative prostate cancer staging and postoperative detection of recurrence utilizing the reverse transcriptase polymerase chain reaction (RT-PCR). J Urol. 1998; 159(5) suppl: 289, A1115.
102. van Nguyen C, Song W, Scardino PT, Wheeler TM, Kattan MW, Slawin KM. RT-PCR for PSA and hK2: implications for staging and patient management in men undergoing radical prostatectomy. J Urol. 1998; 159 (5) suppl: 289, A1114.
103. Gao CL, Maheshwari S, Dean RC, Tatum L, Mooneyhan R, Connelly RR, McLeod DG, Srivastava S, Moul JW. Blinded evaluation of reverse transcriptase-polymerase

chain reaction prostate-specific antigen peripheral blood assay for molecular staging of prostate cancer. Urology. 1999; 53: 714–721.
104. Laribi A, Berteau P, Gala J, Eschwege P, Benoit G, Tombal B, Schmitt F, Loric S. Blood-borne RT-PCR assay for prostasin- specific transcripts to identify circulating prostate cells in cancer patients. Eur Urol. 2001; 39: 65–71.
105. Yu JX, Chao L, Chao J. Prostasin is a novel human serine proteinase from seminal fluid. Purification, tissue distribution, and localization in prostate gland. J Biol Chem. 1994; 269: 18843–18848.
106. Yu JX, Chao L, Chao J. Molecular cloning, tissue-specific expression, and cellular localization of human prostasin mRNA. J Biol Chem. 1995; 270: 13483–13489.
107. Yu JX, Chao L, Ward DC, Chao J. Structure and chromosomal localization of the human prostasin (PRSS8) gene. Genomics. 1996; 32: 334–340.
108. Meijerink J, Mandigers C, van de LL, Tonnissen E, Goodsaid F, Raemaekers J. A novel method to compensate for different amplification efficiencies between patient DNA samples in quantitative real-time PCR. J Mol Diagn. 2001; 3: 55–61.
109. Ylikoski A, Sjoroos M, Lundwall A, Karp M, Lovgren T, Lilja H, Iitia, A. Quantitative reverse transcription-PCR assay with an internal standard for the detection of prostate-specific antigen mRNA. Clin Chem. 1999; 45: 1397–1407.
110. Ylikoski A, Karp M, Pettersson K, Lilja H, Lovgren T. Simultaneous quantification of human glandular kallikrein 2 and prostate-specific antigen mRNAs in peripheral blood from prostate cancer patients. J Mol Diagn. 2001; 3: 111–122.
111. Ylikoski A, Karp M, Lilja H, Lovgren T. Dual-label detection of amplified products in quantitative RT-PCR assay using lanthanide-labeled probes. Biotechniques. 2001; 30: 832–836, 838, 840.
112. Arfman EW, Gustafson K, Schafer S, Williams EA, Nelson PS, Vessella RL. Isolation by magnetic cell sorting of circulating prostate carcinoma cells in peripheral blood and bone marrow. Cancer Res. 2000; 41 suppl: 316, A2009.
113. Gauthier LR, Granotier C, Soria JC, Faivre S, Boige V, Raymond E, Boussin FD. Detection of circulating carcinoma cells by telomerase activity. Brit J Cancer. 2001; 84: 631–635.
114. Sabile A, Louha M, Bonte E, Poussin K, Vona G, Mejean A, Chretien Y, Bougas L, Lacour B, Capron F, Roseto A, Brechot C, Paterlini-Brechot P. Efficiency of Ber-EP4 antibody for isolating circulating epithelial tumor cells before RT-PCR detection. Am J Clin Pathol. 1999; 112: 171–178.
115. Soria JC, Gauthier LR, Raymond E, Granotier C, Morat L, Armand JP, Boussin FD, Sabatier L. Molecular detection of telomerase-positive circulating epithelial cells in metastatic breast cancer patients. Clin Cancer Res. 1999; 5: 971–975.
116. Rosenberg R, Nekarda H, Thorban S, Dahm M, Phelps R, Siewert JR. New density centrifugation method for the enrichment of disseminated tumor cells from peripheral blood. Preliminary results from gastrointestinal cancer patients. Micrometastasis meeting, Hamburg, Germany 2001.
117. Böckmann B, Grill HJ, Giesing M. Molecular characterization of minimal residual cancer cells in patients with solid tumors. Biomol Eng. 2001; 17: 95–111.
118. Colli JL, Ellis WJ, Arfman EW, Lange PH, Vessella RL. The detection and isolation of prostate cancer cells from peripheral blood and bone marrow. J Urol. 2001; 165(5) suppl: 233, A960.
119. Martin VM, Siewert C, Scharl A, Harms T, Heinze R, Ohl S, Radbruch A, Miltenyi S, Schmitz J. Immunomagnetic enrichment of disseminated epithelial tumor cells from peripheral blood by MACS. Exp Hematol. 1998; 26: 252–264.

120. Lansdorp PM, Thomas TE. Purification and analysis of bispecific tetrameric antibody complexes. Mol Immunol. 1990; 27: 659–666.
121. Moldenhauer G, Momburg F, Moller P, Schwartz R, Hammerling GJ. Epithelium-specific surface glycoprotein of Mr 34,000 is a widely distributed human carcinoma marker. Brit J Cancer. 1987; 56: 714–721.
122. Leinung S, Wurl P, Weiss CL, Roder I, Schonfelder M. Cytokeratin-positive cells in bone marrow in comparison with other prognostic factors in colon carcinoma. Langenbecks Arch Surg. 2000; 385: 337–343.
123. Latza U, Niedobitek G, Schwarting R, Nekarda H, Stein H. Ber-EP4: new monoclonal antibody which distinguishes epithelia from mesothelial. J Clin Pathol. 1990; 43: 213–219.
124. Helfrich W, ten Poele R, Meersma GJ, Mulder NH, de Vries EG, de Leij L, Smit EF. A quantitative reverse transcriptase polymerase chain reaction-based assay to detect carcinoma cells in peripheral blood. Brit J Cancer. 1997; 76: 29–35.
125. Vona G, Sabile A, Louha M, Sitruk V, Romana S, Schutze K, Capron F, Franco D, Pazzagli M, Vekemans M, Lacour B, Brechot C, Paterlini-Brechot P. Isolation by size of epithelial tumor cells : a new method for the immunomorphological and molecular characterization of circulating tumor cells. Am J Pathol. 2000; 156: 57–63.
126. Brail LH, Jang A, Billia F, Iscove NN, Klamut HJ, Hill RP. Gene expression in individual cells: analysis using global single cell reverse transcription polymerase chain reaction (GSC RT-PCR). Mutat Res. 1999; 406: 45–54.
127. Harbeck MC, Louie DC, Howland J, Wolf BA, Rothenberg PL. Expression of insulin receptor mRNA and insulin receptor substrate 1 in pancreatic islet beta-cells. Diabetes. 1996; 45: 711–717.
128. Jena PK, Liu AH, Smith DS, Wysocki LJ. Amplification of genes, single transcripts and cDNA libraries from one cell and direct sequence analysis of amplified products derived from one molecule. J Immunol Methods. 1996; 190: 199–213.
129. Roudier MP, True LD, Higano CS, Ellis WJ, Lange PH, Vessella RL. Functional and clonal heterogeneity of bone metastatic prostate cancer. J Urol. 2001; 165(5) suppl: 291, A1199.
130. Pantel K, von Knebel DM. Detection and clinical relevance of micrometastatic cancer cells. Curr Opin Oncol. 2000; 12: 95–101.
131. von Knebel DM, Lacroix J. Nucleic acid based techniques for the detection of rare cancer cells in clinical samples. Cancer Metastasis Rev. 1999; 18: 43–64.
132. Sanchez-Cespedes M, Esteller M, Hibi K, Cope FO, Westra WH, Piantadosi S, Herman JG, Jen J, Sidransky D. Molecular detection of neoplastic cells in lymph nodes of metastatic colorectal cancer patients predicts recurrence. Clin Cancer Res. 1999; 5: 2450–2454.
133. Hayashi N, Arakawa H, Nagase H, Yanagisawa A, Kato Y, Ohta H, Takano S, Ogawa M, Nakamura Y. Genetic diagnosis identifies occult lymph node metastases undetectable by the histopathological method. Cancer Res. 1994; 54: 3853–3856.
134. Hayashi N, Ito I, Yanagisawa A, Kato Y, Nakamori S, Imaoka S, Watanabe H, Ogawa M, Nakamura Y. Genetic diagnosis of lymph-node metastasis in colorectal cancer. Lancet. 1995; 345: 1257–1259.
135. Mao L, Schoenberg MP, Scicchitano M, Erozan YS, Merlo A, Schwab D, Sidransky D. Molecular detection of primary bladder cancer by microsatellite analysis. Science. 1996; 271: 659–662.
136. Behn M, Schuermann M. Sensitive detection of p53 gene mutations by a 'mutant enriched' PCR-SSCP technique. Nucleic Acids Res. 1998; 26: 1356–1358.

137. Somers VA, Pietersen AM, Theunissen PH, Thunnissen FB. Detection of K-ras point mutations in sputum from patients with adenocarcinoma of the lung by point-EXACCT. J Clin Oncol. 1998; 16: 3061–3068.
138. Ahrendt SA, Chow JT, Xu LH, Yang SC, Eisenberger CF, Esteller M, Herman JG, Wu L, Decker PA, Jen J, Sidransky D. Molecular detection of tumor cells in bronchoalveolar lavage fluid from patients with early stage lung cancer. J Natl Cancer Inst. 1999; 91: 332–339.
139. Takeda S, Ichii S, Nakamura Y. Detection of K-ras mutation in sputum by mutant-allele-specific amplification (MASA). Hum Mutat. 1993; 2: 112–117.
140. Austrup F, Uciechowski P, Eder C, Bockmann B, Suchy B, Driesel G, Jackel S, Kusiak I, Grill HJ, Giesing M. Prognostic value of genomic alterations in minimal residual cancer cells purified from the blood of breast cancer patients. Brit J Cancer. 2000; 83: 1664–1673.
141. Lin B, Ferguson C, White JT, Wang S, Vessella R, True LD, Hood L, Nelson PS. Prostate-localized and androgen-regulated expression of the membrane-bound serine protease TMPRSS2. Cancer Res. 1999; 59: 4180–4184.
142. Lin B, White JT, Ferguson C, Bumgarner R, Friedman C, Trask B, Ellis W, Lange P, Hood L, Nelson PS. PART-1: a novel human prostate-specific, androgen-regulated gene that maps to chromosome 5q12. Cancer Res. 2000; 60: 858–863.
143. Lin B, White JT, Ferguson C, Wang S, Vessella R, Bumgarner R, True LD, Hood L, Nelson PS. Prostate short-chain dehydrogenase reductase 1 (PSDR1): a new member of the short-chain steroid dehydrogenase/reductase family highly expressed in normal and neoplastic prostate epithelium. Cancer Res. 2001; 61: 1611–1618.
144. Klein CA, Schmidt-Kittler O, Schardt JA, Pantel K, Speicher MR, Riethmuller G. Comparative genomic hybridization, loss of heterozygosity, and DNA sequence analysis of single cells. Proc Natl Acad Sci USA. 1999; 96: 4494–4499.
145. Hodgson G, Hager JH, Volik S, Hariono S, Wernick M, Moore D, Nowak N, Albertson DG, Pinkel D, Collins C, Hanahan D, Gray JW. Genome scanning with array CGH delineates regional alterations in mouse islet carcinomas. Nat Genet. 2001; 29: 459–464.

Chapter 6

EARLY DISSEMINATED TUMOUR CELLS IN OPERABLE NON-SMALL CELL LUNG CANCER

Bernward Passlick

Department of Surgery, Division of Thoracic Surgery, University of Munich, Germany

Abstract

Metastasis to lymph nodes or distant organs is a well-known feature of poor prognosis in potentially resectable non-small cell lung cancer (NSCLC). However, a significant number of lymph node negative patients die early of metastatic disease. Therefore, it has to be assumed that in some patients an early tumour cell dissemination has occurred which is clearly underestimated by current staging procedures. Recently, it has been shown, that an early dissemination of individual carcinoma cells to regional lymph nodes or bone marrow can be detected by using sensitive immunocytochemical techniques with monoclonal antibodies against epithelium-specific proteins. The incidence of immunohistochemically positive patients varies between 30% and 70% depending on the type of primary tumour, the immunohistochemical staining procedure used and especially on the primary monoclonal antibody. The detection of disseminated tumour cells in lymph nodes or bone marrow by immunocytochemistry is associated with a poorer prognosis in lung cancer. In conclusion, the immunohistochemical detection of early disseminated tumour cells in lymph nodes or bone marrow can help to obtain a more exact identification of patients with an unfavorable prognosis. Whether the identified patients will gain from an adjuvant therapy needs to be evaluated in further studies.

INTRODUCTION

The dissemination of malignant cells to distant organs via lymph nodes or blood vessels in solid tumours can occur at an early stage of primary tumour growth and is regularly underestimated by currently available clinical and pathological staging procedures (1). For example, approximately 40% of patients who undergo surgical resection of non-small cell lung cancer (NSCLC) without overt metastases (pT_{1-2}, N_0, M_0, R_0) relapse within 24 months after surgery (2). This is also reflected in a poor 5-year survival rate of about 60% and suggests that an occult tumour load is the major reason for the high mortality in surgically treated lung cancer patients (3).

Indeed, several groups, including ours, have shown that the early dissemination of individual lung carcinoma cells to regional lymph nodes (4–6) and

K. Pantel (ed.), Micrometastasis, 117–125.

distant organs like the bone marrow (7–9) can be detected by immunocytochemical techniques using monoclonal antibodies against epithelium-specific proteins. In bone marrow the occurrence of cytokeratin-positive cells has recently demonstrated to be indicative for a later clinical relapse (7–9) and the malignant nature of these cells has further been supported by their tumour-associated genetic characteristics and their metastatic capacity after transplantation in immunodeficient mice (10).

DETECTION OF TUMOUR CELLS IN LYMPH NODES

Methodological Aspects

Minimal tumour cell dissemination to regional lymph nodes has been previously assessed by serial sectioning of lymph nodes hematoxylin-eosin (HE) staining and routine histopathologic examination of an extensive number of consecutive sections (11). Using this approach the number of positive lymph nodes can be increased in about 8% to 30% of the specimens (12). However, the method is time-consuming and thus not practicable as a routine procedure for tumour staging. Thus, sensitive immunocytochemical assays with antibodies to epithelial antigens might be more reasonable alternatives.

Monoclonal antibodies to epithelial cytokeratins have been successfully used to identify individual metastatic cells in bone marrow of patients with various epithelial tumours (13). However, since reticulum cells express cytokeratins (14, 15), antibodies directed against these proteins are not the best choice for the identification of individual carcinoma cells in lymph nodes, because somewhat subjective morphological criteria must be imposed.

To develop an observer-independent assay solely based on the assessment of immunoreactivity we used mAb Ber-EP4 for the detection of micrometastatic tumour cells. Ber-EP4 (IgG1; Dako, Hamburg, Germany) is directed against two glycopolypeptides of 34 and 49 kD present on the surface and in the cytoplasm of all epithelial cells except the superficial layers of squamous epithelia, hepatocytes, and parietal cells (16, 17). The antibody does not react with mesenchymal tissue, including lymphoid tissue (16), and can also be used on paraffin sections.

The high sensitivity of mAb Ber-Ep4 for detection of NSCLC cells was supported by positive staining of 81 out of 82 (99%) primary tumours (45 adenocarcinomas and 37 squamous cell carcinomas). The majority of these samples (73/81) displayed a homogeneous staining. The consistent staining of 15 lymph nodes with overt metastases (Stage N_1) further indicated that the corresponding antigens remain preserved during the process of metastases (6).

In order to compare the effectiveness of the immunohistochemical analyses directly with the conventional HE-method two additional sections consecutive to those displaying Ber-Ep4 positive cells were studied. One section was stained by routine HE staining, the other was immunostained with Ber-Ep4. Both sections were then compared with the original positive section by an experienced pathologist without having knowledge of the initial results. Repeated immunostaining resulted in a redetection of Ber-Ep4 positive cells in a neighbouring section in 93.3% of the nodes and in 90.9% of the patients, respectively (6). In our studies on early lymph node dissemination in lung cancer 4–6 m cryostat sections were cut from three different levels of each lymph node. One section per level was stained with the alkaline phosphatase anti-alkaline phosphatase (APAAP)-technique.

Detection Rate and Prognostic Significance

In NSCLC the immunohistochemical staining with the monoclonal antibody Ber-Ep4 revealed disseminated epithelial cells in 35 (6.2%) of 565 lymph nodes that were negative by routine histopathology and 27 (21.6%) of 125 patients with resectable NSCLC (Table 1). These cells occurred as either isolated, single cells or as cell cluster up to three cells present in the sinuses (60%) and the lymphoid tissue of the node (40%). A single positive finding of isolated tumour cells in one section of one lymph node of the investigated patient was a rare event. In 80% of cases, minimal tumour cell spread was found in more than one of the three lymph node sections (31%) or more than one lymph node (55%).

Table 1. Presence of isolated tumour cells in lymph nodes of NSCLC patients*

	Number of Patients Per Group	Number of Patients with Isolated Tumour Cells in Lymph Nodes
Total	125	27 (21.6%)
pT-status		
pT_{1-2}	104	23 (22.1%)
pT_{3-4}	21	4 (19.0%)
pN-status		
pN_0	70	11 (15.7%)
pN_1	25	4 (16.0%)
pN_2	30	12 (40.0%)
pN_{1+2}	55	16 (29.1%)‡
Histological type		
Adenocarcinoma	55	13 (23.6%)
Squamous-cell carcinoma	52	10 (19.2%)
Miscellaneous†	18	4 (22.2%)

Notes

* Modified from (24).

†Adenosquamous carcinoma ($n = 6$) and large cell carcinoma ($n = 12$).

‡ $p = 0.019$ (pN_0 versus pN_{1-2} patients, χ^2-test).

By conventional histopathology, 70 of 125 patients were staged as having pN_0 disease and 55 as pN_{1-2} disease according to the International Union Against Cancer TNM classification (Table 1). In pN_{1-2} patients immunohistochemical staining exposed tumour cell dissemination to resected lymph nodes in 16 cases (29.1%). This was clearly higher in comparison with pN_0 patients, who had Ber-EP4 positive cells in their lymph nodes in 11 cases (15.7%) ($p = 0.019$). Other pathological parameters were not associated with an increased rate of disseminated tumour cells in univariate analysis.

These rates are considerably lower than the frequencies obtained in a recent retrospective study (4), in which 17% of the lymph nodes and 63% of the patients analysed were judged as positive. This discrepancy may in part reflect an increased rate of false-positive findings in the latter study due to the use of a polyclonal anti-keratin antiserum, which may also explain the failure to obtain a prognostic significance.

Our study on NSCLC patients revealed that after an observation time of 64 months, patients with immunohistochemically proven disseminated tumour cells in regional lymph nodes had a significantly reduced overall survival ($p = 0.0001$; Table 2, univariate analysis). Correspondingly, patients with disseminated tumour cells experienced a higher rate of disease relapse than patients without such cells ($p < 0.0001$). Because of the elevated frequency of Ber-EP4 positive cells in higher pN stages (Table 1), a stratification for pN stage was done. In pN_0 disease, patients with disseminated tumour cells had a significant overall survival disadvantage over those without disseminated tumour cells ($p = 0.010$). In pN_{1-2} disease the overall survival rate was also definitely reduced in the presence of

Table 2. Prognostic significance of disseminated tumour cells in lymph nodes in 125 NSCLC patients (uni- and multivariate statistics of overall survival)*

		Multivariate analysis (Cox model)			
Variable	Univariate *p*-value†	Estimated Coefficient	SE	*p*-value	Relative Risk (95% CI)
Lymphatic tumour cell dissemination (positive vs negative)	0.0001	0.935	0.300	0.002	2.5 (1.4–4.6)
pT stage (pT_{1-2} vs pT_{3-4})	0.002	0.602	0.350	0.068	1.8 (0.9–3.6)
pN stage (pN_0 vs pN_{1-2})	0.0001	0.824	0.234	0.011	2.3 (1.2–4.3)
Age (years) (≤ 60 vs > 60)	0.075	0.518	0.294	0.078	1.7 (0.9–3.0)

Notes

* Modified from (24).

† Log-rank test.

these cells and the impact of minimal tumour cell spread on overall survival was comparably strong ($p = 0.027$).

A Cox regression model was applied to analyse the influence of lymphatic tumour cell dissemination, pT stage, pN stage and age on overall survival. The multivariate analysis showed a 2.5 times increased risk for shorter survival and a 2.7 times increased risk for tumour relapse in patients with disseminated tumour cells versus patients without such cells. Pathological N stage had a prognostic value for reduced survival in the same range (relative risk 2.3).

DETECTION OF TUMOUR CELLS IN BONE MARROW

Methodological Aspects

At the time of surgery, we collected tumour samples and bone marrow aspirates from 139 consecutive patients with operable NSCLC who had been treated by lobectomy or pneumectomy in combination with systematic mediastinal lymphadenectomy. Only patients in TNM stage M_0 (i.e., no diagnostic sign for distant metastasis) with completely resected (R_0) primary tumours as assessed by histopathological examination were admitted to the study.

At the primary operation two to four bone marrow aspirates from both sites of the iliac crest and at least one of the ribs were taken through an aspiration needle. By Ficoll-Hypaque density gradient, between 5×10^6 and 6×10^7 (mean 2.5×10^7) mononuclear cells could be isolated out of 2 to 10 mL (mean 5 mL) volume of the aspirates. A defined number of these cells (8×10^4) were then put on glass slides by cytocentrifugation and an immunocytochemical staining was performed using the monoclonal antibody CK2 directed to cytokeratin polypeptide 18 (CK18). CK2 reacts with simple epithelia and tumours derived thereof, as well as most squamous-cell lung carcinomas (18). In our recent immunohistochemical investigation CK18 expression was observed on 95.5% (84/88) of lung tumours (19). For visualization of antibody binding, the APAAP-technique combined with the Neufuchsin method was employed as previously reported (9). The high sensitivity of CK2 for detection of disseminated tumour cells in bone marrow were demonstrated in our previous study (9). There were only 2.8% positive findings in bone marrow aspirates from 215 patients with benign epithelial tumours, non-epithelial neoplasms, and inflammatory diseases or mesenchymal malignancies.

Detection Rate and Prognostic Significance

The immunocytochemical staining with the monoclonal antibody CK2 revealed disseminated epithelial cells in 83 (59.7%) of 139 patients with resectable NSCLC. Frequencies of CK18+ cells were very similar in the different tumour stages (Table 3).

Table 3. Frequency of CK18+ cells in the bone marrow of NSCLC patients according to the tumour stage*

Tumour stage	No. of patients	No. of patients with CK18+ cells in bone marrow (%)
All patients	139	83 (59.7)
Stage IA	15	9 (60.0)
Stage IB	47	23 (48.9)
Stage IIA	4	2 (50.0)
Stage IIB	17	12 (70.6)
Stage IIIA	36	25 (69.4)
Stage IIIB	20	12 (60.0)

Note
* Modified from (25).

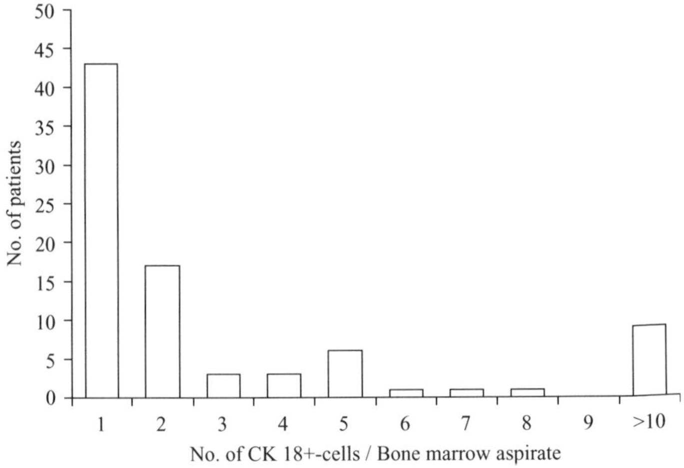

Figure 1. Frequency of CK18+ tumour cells in bone marrow of patients with completely resected NSCLC (modified from (25)).

In patients with pT_1, pN_0 disease ($n = 15$) disseminated tumour cells in the bone marrow were detected in 9 (60%) patients, in pT_2, pN_0 patients ($n = 47$) in 23 (48.9%) cases, and 6 (75%) of the 8 pT_3, pN_0 patients displayed a positive bone marrow status. The CK18+ cells predominantly occurred as isolated cells. Tumour cell clusters were only seen in few cases (10.1% of NSCLC patients) (9). The median number of CK18 positive cells per 4×10^5 mononuclear cells was 2 (range 1–531) (Figure 1). With regard to the total bone marrow, this would be an estimated tumour load of 4×10^6 to 2×10^9 cells (20).

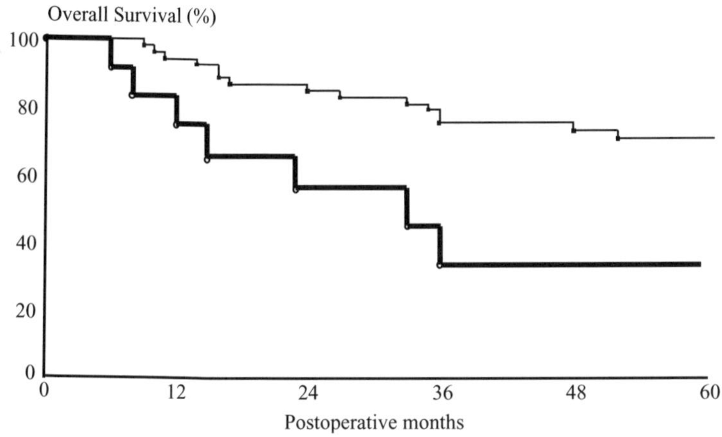

Figure 2. Overall survival (Kaplan-Meier analysis) in pN_O-patients ($n = 66$) with surgically resected NSCLC depending on the presence (—) or absence (—) of immunocytochemically CK18+ tumour cells (≥2 cells per 4×10^5) in bone marrow. The difference is significant: $p = 0.007$ by log-rank test (modified from (25)).

After a median observation time of 66 months, the prognosis of 62 patients with lymph node metastases (pN_{1-2}) was independent of the initial immunocytochemical bone marrow finding. In contrast, in pN_0 disease the patients displaying ≥2 CK18+ tumour cells in bone marrow had a significant overall survival disadvantage over those without isolated tumour cells ($p = 0.007$) (Figure 2). Correspondingly, patients with CK18-positive cells experienced a higher rate of disease relapse than patients without such cells ($p = 0.005$). However, in patients in which only one CK18+ cell was detected in one of the bone marrow aspirates, the prognosis was not statistically different from patients with completely negative bone marrow.

Interestingly, metastatic relapse involving bone or bone marrow was not significantly influenced by the bone marrow status: 7.5% of the patients with negative bone marrow developed bone metastases as compared to 13.3% of the patients with disseminated tumour cells in the bone marrow. A multivariate analysis showed a 2.8 times increased risk for shorter survival in patients with CK18-positive tumour cells versus patients without such cells.

CONCLUSION

In conclusion, the immunohistochemical detection of disseminated tumour cells in bone marrow or lymph nodes can help to obtain a more exact identification of patients with an unfavourable prognosis. These findings provide further support for the suggestion of the standardization committee of the International Union

Against Cancer (UICC) to introduce this early stage of metastatic disease as the category pM1(i) into the existing tumour classification (21). Whether the identified patients will gain from an adjuvant therapy has to be evaluated in further studies. Since most of the disseminated tumour cells appear to be in a dormant (i.e., non-proliferating) state (22), immunotherapeutic approaches might be an alternative to S-phase-specific chemotherapeutic agents. In this context, the EpCam antigen appears to be an interesting target because of its expression on a variety of different epithelia tumour cells, including NSCLC cells (23).

REFERENCES

1. Pantel K, Riethmüller G. Micrometastasis detection and treatment with monoclonal antibodies. Curr Top Microbiol Immunol. 1996;213:1–18.
2. Mountain CF. Revisions in the international system for staging lung cancer. Chest. 1997;111:1710–17.
3. Passlick B, Pantel K. Prognostic factors in stage I non-small cell lung cancer. Zentralbl Chir. 1996;121:851–60.
4. Chen ZL, Perez S, Holmes CE, Wang HJ, Coulson WF, Wen DR, Cochran AJ. Frequency and distribution of occult micrometastases in lymph nodes of patients with non-small cell lung cancer. J Natl Cancer Inst. 1993;85:493–8.
5. Maruyama R, Sugio K, Mitsodomi T, Saitoh G, Ishida T, Sugimachi K. Relationship between early recurrence and micrometastases in the lymph nodes of patients with stage I non-small cell lung cancer. J Thorac Cardiovas Surg. 1997;114:535–43.
6. Passlick B, Izbicki JR, Kubuschok B, Nathrath W, Thetter O, Pichlmeier U, Schweiberer L, Riethmüller G, Pantel K. Immunohistochemical assessment of individual tumour cells in lymph nodes of patients with non-small cell lung cancer. J Clin Oncol. 1994;12:1827–32.
7. Cote RJ, Beattie EJ, Chaiwun B, Shi SR, Harvey J, Chen SC, Sherrod AE, Groshen S, Taylor CR. Detection of occult bone marrow micrometastases in patients with operable lung carcinoma. Ann Surg. 1995;222:415–25.
8. Ohgami A, Mitsodomi T, Sugio K, Tsuda T, Oyama T, Nishida K, Osaki T, Yasumoto K. Micrometastatic tumour cells in the bone marrow of patients with non-small cell lung cancer. Ann Thorac Surg. 1997;64:363–7.
9. Pantel K, Izbicki JR, Passlick B, Angstwurm M, Häussinger K, Thetter O, Riethmüller G. Frequency and prognostic significance of isolated tumour cells detected in bone marrow of non-small cell lung cancer patients without overt metastases. Lancet. 1996;347:649–53.
10. Pantel K, Dickmanns A, Zippelius F, Klein Ch, Hoechtelen-Vollmar B, Schlimok G, Weckermann D, Oberneder R, Shi J, Fanning E *et al.* Establishment of carcinoma cell lines from bone marrow of patients with minimal residual cancer: a novel source of tumor cell vaccines. J Natl Cancer Inst. 1995;87:1162–8.
11. International Breast Cancer Study Group. Prognostic significance of occult axillary lymph node micrometastases from breast cancers. Lancet. 1990;335:1565–8.
12. Dowlatshahi K, Fan M, Snider HC, Habib FA. Lymph node micrometastases from breast carcinoma: reviewing the dilemma. Cancer. 1997;80:1188–97.
13. Pantel K, Braun S, Passlick B, Schlimok G. Minimal residual epithelial cancer: diagnostic approaches and prognostic relevance. Prog Hstochem Cytochem. 1996;30:1–46.

14. Domagala W, Bedner E, Chosia M, Weber K, Osborn M. Keratin-positive reticulum cells in fine needle aspirates and touch imprints of hyperplastic lymph nodes. Acta Cytol. 1991;36:241–5.
15. Doglioni C, Dell'Orto P, Zanetti G, Iuzzolino P, Coggi G, Viale G. Cytokeratin-immunoreactive cells of human lymph nodes and spleen in normal and pathological conditions. Virchows Archiv A Pathol Anat. 1990;416:479–90.
16. Momburg F, Moldenhauer G, Hämmerling GJ, Möller P. Immunohistochemical study of the expression of a Mr 34,000 human epithelium-specific surface glycoprotein in normal and malignant tissues. Cancer Res. 1987;47:2883–91.
17. Latza U, Niedobitek G, Schwarting R, Nekarda H, Stein H. Ber-EP4: new monoclonal antibody which distinguishes epithelia from mesothelia. J Clin Pathol. 1990;43:213–19.
18. Debus E, Moll R, Franke WW, Weber K, Osborn M. Immunohistochemical distinction of human carcinomas by cytokeratin typing with monoclonal antibodies. Am J Pathol. 1984;114:121–30.
19. Pantel K, Izbicki JR, Angstwurm M, Braun S, Passlick B, Karg O, Thetter O, Riethmüller G. Immunocytological detection of bone marrow micrometastasis in operable non-small cell lung cancer. Cancer Res. 1993;53:1027–31.
20. Harrison WJ. The total cellularity of the bone marrow in man. J Clin Pathol. 1962; 15:254–9.
21. Hermanek P. pTNM and residual tumor classifications: problems of assessment and prognostic significance. World J Surg. 1995;19:184–90.
22. Pantel K, Schlimok G, Braun S, Kutter D, Lindemann F, Schaller G, Funke I, Izbicki JR, Riethmüller G. Differential expression of proliferation-associated molecules in individual micrometastatic carcinoma cells. J Natl Cancer Inst. 1993;85:1419–24.
23. Passlick B, Sienel W, Seen-Hilber R, Wöckel W, Thetter O, Pantel K. The 17-1A antigen is expressed on primary, metastatic and disseminated non-small cell lung carcinoma cells. Int J Cancer. 2000;87:548–52.
24. Kubuschok B, Passlick B, Izbicki JR, Thetter O, Pantel K. Disseminated tumor cells in lymph nodes as a determinant for survival in surgically resected non-small cell lung cancer. J Clin Oncol. 1999;17:19–24.
25. Passlick B, Kubuschok B, Izbicki JR, Thetter O, Pantel K. Isolated tumor cells in bone marrow predict reduced survival in node-negative non-small cell lung cancer. Ann Thorac Surg. 1999;68:2053–8.

Chapter 7

PROGNOSTIC VALUE OF MINIMAL RESIDUAL DISEASE IN ESOPHAGEAL CANCER

Peter Scheuemann, Stefan B. Hosch, Jacob R. Izbicki

Department of General and Thoracic Surgery, Universitätsklinikum Eppendorf, Martinistrasse 52, D-20246 Hamburg, Germany

Abstract

A substantial proportion of patients (40% to 50%) with supposedly localized esophageal cancer who had undergone curative surgical treatment with complete tumour removal suffer from a metastatic tumour relapse within 24 months after surgery. A reason for such an early tumour relapse in these patients might be a minimal tumour cell dissemination (minimal residual disease, MRD) present at the time of operation, which cannot be detected by clinical and routine histopathological tumour staging procedures. Over the past 10 years, more sensitive immunohisto-/-cytochemical and nucleic acid based assays have been developed that are based on the detection of epithelial cell-or tumour-associated marker proteins and are able to detect single tumour cells or small tumour cell clusters present in lymph nodes classified as tumour-free by conventional histopathologic analysis, bone marrow or blood. Here we present an overview of recent studies concerning the prevalence and prognostic value of occult tumour cells in lymph nodes and bone marrow of patients with esophageal cancer identified by antibody or nucleic acid based assays.

INTRODUCTION

Despite advances in early diagnosis and more radical surgical treatment, prognosis of patients with esophageal carcinoma has not changed markedly over the last decades with reported postoperative survival rates of 10% to 36% (1–5). Approximately half of the patients develop early metastatic relapse after complete resection of their apparently localized primary tumours (6). It is therefore assumed that these patients had occult metastases already present at time of primary surgery and undetectable by current tumour staging methods. Over the past 10 years, more sensitive immunohisto-/-cytochemical and nucleic acid based methods have been developed that are based on the detection of epithelial cell-or tumour-associated markers and that are able to detect single tumour cells present in lymph nodes classified as tumour-free by conventional histopathologic analysis (7–14), bone marrow (6, 15–17) or blood (18–21) (see Table 1).

For the immunohisto-/-cytochemical detection of occult epithelial tumour cells in bone marrow and pathohistologically negative lymph nodes, most studies applied cytokeratins (CKs) as marker antigens. These proteins are stably,

K. Pantel (ed.), Micrometastasis, 127–138.

Table 1. Overview of immunhisto-/cytochemical assays used for detection of early disseminated tumour cells

Compartment of Tumour Cell Screening	Detection Antibodies (target proteins)	Detection Rate (%) [pos. LK (%)]	Prognostic Impact	Reference
LN	AE1/AE3 (CK)	20/78 (26) 40/574 (7)	No impact	34
LN	AE1/AE3 (CK)	14/37 (38)	DFS*, OS	38
LN	AE1/AE3 (CK)	15/41 (37)	OS	36
LN	Ber-EP4 (EpCAM)	*42/68 (62) total* *15/30 (50) pN0* [67/399 (17)]	DFS*, OS*	9
LN	Ber-EP4 (EpCAM)	89/126 (71)*total* 30/54 (56)*pN0* [150/634 (23)]	DFS*, OS* DFS*	8
LN	AE1/AE3 (CK)	39/59 (55.5)	OS	37
LN	AE1/AE3 (CK) anti-EMA (EMA)	26/115 (22.6)	Not evaluated	42
LN	AE1/AE3 (CK)	6/18 (33) *pNo* 15/46 (33) *total*	Not evaluated	41
BM	CK2 (CK)	1/8 (12.5)	Not evaluated	32
BM	CK2 (CK) A45-B/B3 (CK) KL1 (CK)	37/90 (41)	DFS, OS	6
BM	A45-B/B3 (CK)	25/68 (37)	No impact	9
BM	A45-B/B3 (CK)	28/79 (35)	DFS, OS	own data (not published)
BM	A45-B/B3 (CK)	29/75 (39)	OS*	31

Notes:

* Prognostic value was confirmed by multivariate analysis. Abbreviations: LN: lymph node; BM: bone marrow; CK: cytokeratin; EMA: epithelial-membrane antigen; DFS: disease-free survival; OS: overall survival.

abundantly and homogeneously expressed in a majority of epithelial tumours, including esophageal carcinoma (22). This extremely sensitive approach is able to detect 1 tumour cell in the background of 1×10^6 normal mononuclear bone marrow or lymph node cells (22). Performing this immunohisto-/-cytochemical approach, occult tumour cell detection rates of 12.5% to 41% for bone marrow and 26% to 56% for lymph nodes of esophageal cancer patients without overt lymph node metastatases (pN0) have been reported. For nucleic acid based tumour cell detection, most studies applied reverse transcriptase polymerase chain reaction (RT-PCR) assays to detect carcinoembryonic antigen (CEA) messenger RNA (mRNA), which is certainly expressed at different levels in a varity of gastrointestinal carcinoma, including esophageal carcinoma, with tumour cell detection rates between 5% and 55% in histopathologically negative lymph nodes.

Although an increasing number of published studies indicates that these early tumour cell deposits, especially in 'tumour-free' lymph nodes, appeared to be strong and independent predictors of tumour relapse in several carcinoma entities (7–10, 12–14, 21, 23, 24), it remains unclear whether these deposits are viable tumour cells with a metastatic potential or shedded tumour cells with a limited lifespan or even simply laboratory artefacts. This scepticism is based upon the observation that immunohistochemically identifiable cells lack sometimes the typical morphology of tumour cells (25). In addition, the specificity of ultrasensitive nucleic acid based molecular assays is limited by the lack of any morphological correlate and the low-level ectopic expression of tumour marker transcripts in the surrounding normal tissues (e.g., CEA mRNA in normal lymphoid tissue) (26–28). As a consequence, the detection of micrometastases with these new methods has not been incorporated in the current UICC tumour staging nomenclature (29).

IMMUNOCYTOCHEMICAL DETECTION OF OCCULT TUMOUR CELLS IN BONE MARROW

Thorban *et al.* (6) used three different monoclonal antibodies (mAb) directed against different CK components for occult tumour cell detection in bone marrow: mAb CK2, which recognize CK component 18, mAb KL1, directed against a pan-CK component of 56,000 kDa, and mAb A45-B/B3, which detects a common epitope present on a varity of CK components, including CK8, 18, and 19 (6, 30). Using these mAbs, 6/90 (6.7%), 31/90 (34.4%), and 10/43 (23.3%) patients showed CK-positive cells in their bone marrow applying mAbs CK2, KL1, and A45-B/B3, respectively. Altogether, CK-positive cells were detected in 37 (41%) of 90 bone marrow samples. In 32 of these 37 positive samples, less than 10 CK-positive cells/4×10^5 MNC were found. The relative proportion of CK-positive cells ranged between 1 and 82 CK-positive cells/4×10^5 mononuclear cells (MNC). For postoperative follow-up analyses 42 patients were available. 19 (45%) of these patients had CK-positive cells in their bone marrow. 15/19 patients (79%) with positive marrow findings developed tumour relapse, compared with 3/23 patients with CK-negative bone marrow. Univariate survival analysis revealed that the presence of CK-positive cells in bone marrow predicted for a reduced relapse-free ($p = 0.019$) and overall survival ($p = 0.036$). However, the analysed number of patients – especially for survival analysis where only 42 patients could be included – was very small. Furthermore, univariate significance of CK-positive cells in bone marrow was not confirmed by a multivariate analysis. This was done in a further study by Thorban *et al.* (31), where bone marrow samples of 75 patients were analysed with mAb A45-B/B3. 29 (38.7%) of these patients showed A45-B/B3-positive cells in their bone marrow. In univariate survival analysis, patients with A45-B/B3-positive cells died more frequently and more rapidly compared to patients without these cells ($p < 0.001$). Furthermore, the prognostic impact of CK positivity in bone marrow could be confirmed by a multivariate analysis as the strongest independent prognostic factor beside the T-category.

In contrast, analysing bone marrow aspirates of 68 patients with resectable esophageal carcinoma, our study group could not find any significant correlation between occult tumour cell detection in bone marrow and both relapse-free and overall survival using mAb A45-B/B3. Occult tumour cells were detected in 25 (37%) bone marrow samples. Interestingly, all patients that were found to have A45-B/B3-positive cells in their bone marrow showed immunohistochemically identifiable isolated tumour cells in lymph nodes. However, these results were not confirmed in a later ongoing study were a total of 79 patients with completely resected (R0) esophageal carcinoma were analysed (data not published). Occult tumour cells in bone marrow were detected in 28 (35%) of the 79 patients by mAb A45-B/B3. Postoperative survival analyses with a median observation time of 25 months (range 1–101 months) revealed that patients with A45-B/B3-positive bone marrow cells had both a significantly reduced relapse-free ($p = 0.026$) and overall survival time ($p = 0.015$) compared to patients without these cells. However, prognostic importance of A45-B/B3 positivity in bone marrow could not be confirmed in multivariate analyses, where exclusively pathohistologically proven nodal involvement (pN1) predicted relapse and tumour-related death.

Another immunocytological approach was tested by O'Sullivan *et al.* (32) choosing the technique of flow cytometry for identifying and quantifying micrometastatic tumour cells in bone marrow of patients with different gastrointestinal carcinoma entities, including esophageal carcinoma, using a directly fluorochrome-labelled mAb against CK18. Thereby, a concentration of ≥ 10 CK18-positive cell/1×10^5 normal mononuclear marrow cells was defined as a positive result. A total of 27 (26.5%) of 102 analysed patients was found to have flow cytometric CK18-positive cell in their bone marrow, *inter alia*, 1 of 8 patients with squamous cell carcinoma (SCC) of the esophagus. However, one critical point of this study seems to be the low specificity of flow cytometry, which results in our experience in false positive findings between 0.5% and 3% in specificity controls with non-specific isotype-antibodies. Moreover, lack of specificity is supported by the immunocytochemical analyses where the majority of carcinoma patients have clearly fewer than 10 CK-positive cell/$4 \times 10^5 - 1 \times 10^6$ mononuclear marrow cells (6, 22), compared to 18 (66.7%) patients in the study of O'Sullivan *et al.*, with 10–50 CK-positive cells and 9 (33%) patients with levels of 50 up to 500 CK18-positive cell/1×10^5 normal mononuclear marrow cells.

IMMUNOHISTOCHEMICAL TUMOUR CELL DETECTION IN PATHOHISTOLOGICALLY TUMOUR-FREE LYMPH NODES

Lymph node metastasis is the most important parameter of poor prognosis in a variety of carcinoma entities, including esophageal cancer, when no evidence of systemic metastases is present. Reported relapse rates of 10% within the first 2 postoperative years in patients with UICC stage I esophageal cancer (pT1pN0M0)

(33) leads to the development of improved immunohistochemical techniques to detect occult disseminated tumour cells, especially in lymph nodes. Although it seems obvious that regional tumour spread is clinically important, an increasing number of studies on many tumours, including esophageal cancer (7–10, 12, 21, 23, 24), could demonstrate the prognostic value of immunohistochemically identifiable occult tumour cells in lymph nodes, other investigators have found that detection of these tumour cells is not correlated with a worse clinical outcome (11, 34).

Most studies analysing pathohistologically negative lymph nodes in esophageal cancer used the monoclonal anti-pan-CK antibody AE1/AE3, which is directed against the CK components 1–6, 8, 10, 14–16, and 19 (35). Glickman *et al.* (34) examined 574 'tumour-free' lymph nodes from 49 patients with pN0-adenocarcinoma and 29 patients with pN0-squamous cell carcinoma (SCC) of the esophagus using this mAb. In total, AE1/AE3-positive cells were found in 7% of lymph nodes (40/574) from 20 of 78 patients (26%). However, the presence of CK-positive cells was not correlated significantly with relapse-free or overall survival. In contrast, Natsugoe *et al.* (36) analysed pathohistologically negative nodes from 41 pN0 patients with esophageal squamous cell carcinoma (SCC) using also mAb AE1/AE3. In cases of nodal AE1/AE3 positivity, they made a distinction between real 'micrometastases' (MM), defined as single tumour cells or small tumour cell clusters <0.5 mm in greatest diameter with a surrounding stromal reaction, and tumour cell microinvolvement (TCM), defined as single tumour cells or small tumour cell clusters without this stromal reaction. AE1/AE3-positive MM and AE1/AE3-positive TCM were detected in 13 (31.7%) and 2 (4.9%) cases, respectively. In survival analysis, patients with MM, but not with TCM, showed a significantly reduced survival compared to patients without these cells. However, prognostic impact of these MM were not analysed in a multivariate analysis. Matsumoto *et al.* (37), also distinguishing between TCM and MM, found AE1/AE3 positive MM in 39 (66.1%) of 59 patients with pN0 esophageal SCC. Tumour recurrence was observed in 17 patients (28.8%) and all but one of them had nodal MM. Also 5-year survival rates were significantly poorer in patients with AE1/AE3-positive lymph nodes. Similar to Natsugoe *et al.*, no multivariate survival analysis was done to clarify the independent prognostic impact of occult nodal tumour cells. This was done by Komukai *et al.* (38) analysing pathohistologically negative lymph nodes of 37 patients with pN0 esophageal SCC. AE1/AE3-positive tumour cells were detected in 14 (38%) of these patients and postoperative tumour recurrence was significantly more frequent in patients with occult nodal tumour cells than in those without these cells ($p = 0.008$). Survival analyses revealed that the AE1/AE3-positive patients had a significantly shorter relapse-free ($p = 0.04$) and overall survival ($p = 0.002$). Furthermore, AE1/AE3-positive tumour cells in lymph nodes had an independent prognostic importance for relapse-free survival by multivariate analysis.

Another study that could demonstrate the independent prognostic value of immunohistochemically identifiable tumour cells in lymph nodes in esophageal cancer was done by our group (9). In this study, 399 pathohistologically negative lymph nodes obtained from 68 patients were analysed using the anti-epithelial mAb Ber-EP4, which is directed against two glycoproteins of 34 and 49 kDa on the cell surface of epithelial cells (39). Prior studies on esophageal primary tumours and pathohistologically identified lymph node metastases could demonstrate that Ber-EP4 was consistent immunoreactive in all lesions analysed. Furthermore, no Ber-EP4 staining was found in a series of lymph nodes from 24 patients with malignant mesenchymal tumours or benign disorders. In contrast to anti-CK antibodies, which can react with CK expressing normal reticuloendothelial cell (40), mAb Ber-EP4 showed no reaction with these cells. Ber-EP4-positive tumour cells were found in 67 (17%) of the 399 pathohistologically negative nodes obtained from 42 (62%) of the 68 patients. Fifteen of 30 patients staged as pN0 and 27 of 38 patients staged as pN1 showed Ber-EP4 positive cells in their pathohistologically 'tumour-free' lymph nodes. In survival analyses, both pN0 ($p = 0.01$) and pN1 patients ($p = 0.007$) had a significantly reduced relapse-free survival when occult nodal tumour cells were detected. Furthermore, independent of the pathohistological lymph node status Ber-EP4-positive cells found in tumour-free nodes were independently predictive of significantly reduced relapse-free (0.008) and overall survival ($p = 0.03$). These results could be confirmed in a later ongoing study. We analysed 126 patients with completely resectable esophageal cancer, and also here we provide evidence for a strong and independent prognostic influence of immunohistochemically identifiable tumour cells in apparently 'tumour-free' lymph nodes (8). A total of 634 lymph nodes classified as free of metastases were further examined immunohistochemically. Ber-EP4 expressing isolated tumour cells were identified in 150 (23%) of these 634 pathohistologically negative nodes from 89 (71%) patients. Thirty (34%) of these patients were staged as pN0, and 59 (66%) patients were staged as pN1. In the group of 54 patients classified as pN0 immunohistochemical analyses revealed mAb Ber-EP4-positive cells in 30 (56%) patients.

For survival analysis 48 of these patients were available: 28 (58%) of them were found to have Ber-EP4-positive cells in their lymph nodes. These patients had a median relapse-free survival of 27 months compared to >55 months in the 20 Ber-EP4-negative pN0 patients ($p = 0.005$). Moreover, 10 of 28 patients with Ber-EP4-positive cells relapsed and 9 of these patients died during the observation period in contrast to one of 20 Ber-EP4-negative pN0 patients that developed recurrence and died. Multivariate survival analysis underlined the strong and independent prognostic significance of Ber-EP4-positive cells in these 'node-negative' (pN0) patients ($p = 0.01$). In patients with a histopathological pN1 stage no significant difference between Ber-EP4-positive and -negative patients could be revealed for median relapse-free (6 months versus 17 months, $p = 0.28$) or overall survival (10 months versus 18 months, $p = 0.24$). Combining the data for all surviving patients with a median observation time of 21 months (range 6–83), the presence of Ber-EP4-positive cells in tumour-free lymph nodes was associated with a significantly decreased relapse-free survival (56 months for patients without Ber-EP4-positive cells versus 11 months for patients with Ber-EP4-positive cells, $p = 0.002$). Multivariate Cox regression analysis revealed an independent prognostic influence of immunohistochemically detectable tumour cells in lymph nodes for both relapse-free ($p = 0.01$) and overall survival ($p = 0.02$).

Another study by Bonavina *et al.* (41) examined retrospectively 1,301 pathohistologically negative nodes from 46 patients with adenocarcinoma of the esophagogastric junction with mAb (AE1/AE3). In one third of the patients CK-positive tumour cells could be found by immunohistochemical reexamination. Six of 18 patients previously considered pN0 showed occult tumour cells in their lymph nodes, and 3 of these 6 patients had developed tumour recurrence. A similar approach was performed by Chen *et al.* (42) that reexamined retrospectively paraffin-embedded samples of pathohistologically negative lymph nodes of 115 UICC stage I esophageal carcinoma patients using mAbs AE1/AE3 and anti-EMA, directed against the epithelial membrane antigen. Occult nodal tumour cells were identified in 26 (22.6%) of the 115 patients.

NUCLEIC ACID-BASED APPROACHES

Although most investigators demonstrated specificity of their nucleic acid-based tumour cell detection assays via exclusion of false positive marker transcript detection in prior analyses of lymph node or bone marrow samples from patients with benign disorders, described detection of low-level ectopic expression of tumour marker transcripts in surrounding normal tissues (e.g., CEA mRNA in normal lymphoid tissue (26–28) or cytokeratin mRNA in non-epithelial cells (43, 44)) demonstrates limitation of these approaches. Nevertheless, an increasing number of studies using molecular techniques for screening of early disseminated tumour cells in bone marrow or lymph nodes has been published in the last years (see Table 2).

Table 2. Overview of nucleic acid based assays used for detection of early disseminated tumour cells

Compartment of Tumour Cell Screening	Marker mRNAs	Detection Rate pos. Pat. (%) [pos.LK (%)]	Prognostic Impact	Reference
LN	CEA	5/10 (50) [36/73 (49)]	Not evaluated	45
LN	CEA	4/7 (57) [47/87 (54)]	Not evaluated	47
LN	CEA	[17/31(55)]	Not evaluated	46
LN	CEA	6/21 (29) [79/373 (21)]	Not evaluated	48
LN	SCC	[29/584 (5)]	Not evaluated	49

Notes
Prognostic value was confirmed by multivariate analysis. Abbreviations: LN: lymph node; BM: bone marrow; CEA: carcinoembryonic antigen; SCC: squamous cell carcinoma antigen.

Luketich *et al.* (45) examined CEA-mRNA expression on 73 pathohistologically negative lymph nodes from 30 patients with esophageal cancer by RT-PCR. In 36 (49%) of these nodes CEA mRNA was found. Furthermore, 5 of 10 patients pathohistologically staged as pN0 were positive in CEA PT-PCR analysis. Three of these 5 patients with CEA-positive nodes developed recurrence and/or died in course of their disease compared to 1 of 5 patients without CEA-positive nodes with recurrent disease. Kassis *et al.* (46) analysed 31 pathohistologically negative lymph nodes harvested from 13 patients by CEA RT-PCR. In 17 (55%) of these 31 nodes CEA mRNA was detected. Another study examined 87 pathohistologically negative lymph nodes sampled from 13 patients by a CEA-specific RT-PCR assay (47). Sensitivity ratio of the used RT-PCR assay was given with 1 CEA expressing cancer cell in a background of 1×10^5 normal lymphocytes. CEA mRNA was detected in 47 (54%) of 87 histological negative nodes from 13 patients. In routine histopathology lymph node metastases were found in 6 (46%) of these 13 patients compared to 10 (77%) of 13 patients using RT-PCR. Kijima *et al.* (48) examined a total of 373 pathohistologically negative lymph nodes from 21 patients with esophageal cancer also by CEA-specific RT-PCR. Ten of these patients were categorized as pN0, and 11 patients were staged as pN1; 79 (21%) of the 373 pathohistologically negative nodes were found to be positive for CEA mRNA. In 2 and 11 of these 79 nodes occult tumour cells were discovered by histopathological reexamination and immunohistochemical staining procedure, respectively.

Kano *et al.* (49) used a RT-nested PCR against the squamous carcinoma (SCC) antigen transcript to detect occult nodal tumour cells in esophageal SCC patients. This SCC antigen, widely known as a serum tumour marker, was reported as a target gene for detection of disseminated tumour cells in peripheral blood in cervical cancer. In this study, a total of 584 pathohistologically negative lymph nodes from 14 esophageal SCC patients were analysed by RT-PCR against SCC mRNA. Sensitivity ratio of the used RT-PCR assay was 100 SCC expressing tumour cells in a background of 1×10^7 normal peripheral blood mononucleocytes and no SCC mRNA expression was found in prior analysis of 43 control lymph nodes from patients with non-malignant disorders. Occult nodal tumour cells were identified in 29 (5%) of the 584 nodes.

However, in view of the extremely low number of analysed patients, no further evaluation of patient outcome was performed in these five studies and, therefore, clinical importance of tumour marker transcript detection in pathohistologically negative lymph nodes of esophageal cancer patients has to be clarified in further studies with larger numbers of patients.

CONCLUSION

Despite the progress made in clinical and surgical oncology in recent decades, the prognosis of patients with resectable esophageal carcinoma is still limited by metastatic relapse (50) which indicates an early tumour cell spread at the time of surgery.

This tumour cell spread is not detectable by conventional tumour-staging methods and, therefore, reliable information about the individual risk to develop recurrence is not available by means of these methods particularly in patients with early-stage cancer. Therefore, new parameters are needed for the identification of patients at a high risk of tumour recurrence, which cannot be cured by surgery alone, but needs further adjuvant treatment. The detection of the earliest manifestations of tumour cell dissemination with mAbs seems to be a promising approach which might enable us to identify suitable candidates for adjuvant strategies. The clinical importance of tumour marker transcript detection in histopathologically negative lymph nodes of esophageal cancer patients has to be proven in further studies with larger numbers of patients. In the last 10 years, new immunologic and molecular analytical procedures have been developed to diagnose and characterize minimal residual cancer. Standardization of the applied methods are needed before their introduction into routine clinical use. Therefore, studies are currently in progress to evaluate and standardize these protocols (51). The encouraging results from studies on the prognostic relevance of disseminated tumour cells in different compartments (lymph nodes, bone marrow) have led to a first proposal for inclusion into the International Union Against Cancer (UICC) staging classification by Hermanek (29). Thus, additional tumour-staging information could be provided as part of the pathologic assessment process in the TNM classification system. Improved methods for genomic analysis of single tumour cells (52–54) and for assessing target molecule expression may increase the diagnostic precision of current detection techniques, thus optimizing the therapeutic options for the individual patient.

If examination for occult tumour cell spread will be incorporated into future clinical trials for the evaluation of cancer treatments, individually tailored adjuvant therapy seems possible in the future at least for patients with proven residual disease. This would represent a substantial advance in oncologic treatment.

REFERENCES

1. Lerut T, DeLeyn P, Coosemans W, van Raemdonck D, Scheys I, LeSaffre E. Surgical strategies in esophageal carcinoma with emphasis on radical lymphadenectomy. Ann Surg. 1992; 216:583–590.
2. Siewert JR, Bartels H, Bollschweiler E, Dittler HJ, Fink U, Hölscher AH, Roder JD. Plattenepithelcarzinom des Ösophagus: Behandlungskonzept der Chirurgischen Klinik der Technischen Universität München. Chirurg. 1992; 63:693–700.
3. Watanabe H. Plattenepithelcarcinom des Oesophagus. Chirurg. 1992; 63:689–692.
4. Earlam R. Epidemiology of Esophageal Cancer from the European Point of View. In: Siewert JR, Hölscher AH, editors. Diseases of the Esophagus. Berlin, Heidelberg: Springer Verlag, 1988, pp. 11–18.
5. Goldminc M, Maddern G, Le Prise E, Meunier B, Campion JP, Launois B. Oesophagectomy by a transhiatal approach or thoracotomy: a prospective randomized trial. Brit J Surg. 1993; 80:367–370.

6. Thorban S, Roder JD, Nekarda H, Funk A, Siewert JR, Pantel K. Immunocytochemical detection of disseminated tumour cells in bone marrow of patients with esophageal carcinoma. J Natl Cancer Inst. 1996; 88:1222–1227.
7. Hosch SB, Knoefel WT, Metz S, Stoecklein N, Niendorf A, Broelsch CE, Izbicki JR. Early lymphatic tumour cell dissemination in pancreatic cancer: frequency and prognostic significance. Pancreas. 1997; 15:154–159.
8. Hosch SB, Kraus J, Scheunemann P, Izbicki JR, Schneider C, Schumacher U, Witter K, Speicher MR, Pantel K. Malignant potential and prognostic impact of occult disseminated tumour cells in patients with esophageal cancer. Cancer Res. 2000; 60:6836–6840.
9. Izbicki JR, Hosch SB, Pichlmeier U, Rehders A, Busch C, Niendorf A, Passlick B, Broelsch CE, Pantel K. Prognostic value of immunohistochemically identifiable tumour cells in lymph nodes of patients with completely resected esophageal cancer. N Engl J Med. 1997; 337:1188–1194.
10. Pantel K, Braun S, Passlick B, Schlimok G. Minimal residual epithelial cancer: diagnostic approaches and prognostic relevance. Prog Histochem Cytochem. 1996; 30:1–60.
11. Greenson JK, Isenhart CE, Rice R, Mojzisik C, Houchens D, Martin EW. Identification of occult micrometastases in pericolic lymph nodes of Dukes' B colorectal cancer patients using monoclonal antibodies against cytokeratin and CC49. Cancer. 1994; 73:563–569.
12. Calaluce R, Miedema BW, Yesus Y. Micrometastasis in colorectal carcinoma: a review. J Surg Oncol. 1998; 67:194–202.
13. Sidransky E. Nucleic acid-based methods for detection of cancer. Science. 1997; 278:1054–1059.
14. Liefers GJ, Cleton-Janson AM, Van de Velde CJH, Hermans J, Van Krieken JHJM, Cornelissen CJ, Tollenaar AEM. Micrometastases and survival in stage II colorectal cancer. N Engl J Med. 1998; 339:223–228.
15. Lindemann F, Schlimok G, Dirschedl P, Witte J, Riethmuller G. Prognostic significance of micrometastatic tumour cells in bone marrow of colorectal cancer patients. Lancet. 1992; 19:685–691.
16. Maehara Y, Yamamoto M, Oda S, Baba H, Kusumoto T, Ohno S, Ichiyoshi Y, Sugimachi K. Cytokeratin-positive cells in bone marrow for identifying distant micrometastasis of gastric cancer. Brit J Cancer. 1996; 73:83–87.
17. Pantel K, Izbicki JR, Passlick B, Angstwurm M, Häussinger K, Thetter O, Riethmüller G. Frequency and prognostic significance of isolated tumour cells in bone marrow of patients with non-small-cell lung cancer without overt metastases. Lancet. 1996; 347:649–653.
18. Moreno JG, Croce CM, Fischer R, Monne M, Vihko P, Mulholland SG, Gomella LG. Detection of hematogenous micrometastasis in patients with prostate cancer. Cancer Res. 1992; 52:6110–6112.
19. Gudemann CJ, Weitz J, Kienle P, Lacroix J, Wiesel MJ, Soder M, Benner A, Staehler G, Doeberitz MJ. Detection of hematogenous micrometastasis in patients with transitorial cell carcinoma. J Urol. 2000; 164:532–536.
20. Schoenfeld A, Kruger KH, Gomm J, Sinnett HD, Gazet JC, Sacks N, Bender HG, Luqmani Y, Coombes RC. The detection of micrometastases in the peripheral blood and bone marrow of patients with breast cancer using immunohistochemistry and reverse transcriptase polymerase chain reaction for keratin 19. Eur J Cancer. 1997; 33:854–861.
21. Lindblom A. Improved tumour staging in colorectal cancer. N Engl J Med. 1998; 339:264–265.

22. Pantel K, Cote RJ, Fodstad O. Detection and clinical importance of micrometastatic disease. J Natl Cancer Inst. 1999; 91:1313–1324.
23. Passlick B, Izbicki JR, Kubuschok B, Nathrath W, Thetter O, Pichlmeier U, Schweiberer L, Riethmueller G, Pantel K. Immunohistochemical assessment of individual tumour cells in lymph nodes of patients with non-small-cell lung cancer. J Clin Oncol. 1994; 12:1827–1832.
24. Trojani M, de Mascarel I, Bonichon F, Coindre JM, Delsol G. Micrometastases to axillary lymph nodes from carcinoma of breast: detection by immunohistochemistry and prognostic significance. Brit J Cancer. 1987; 55:303–306.
25. Hosch SB, Pantel K, Izbicki JR. Cryptic tumour cells in lymph nodes of patients with esophageal cancer. N Engl J Med. 1998; 338:550.
26. Ko Y, Klinz M, Totzke G, Gouni-Berthold I, Sachinidis A, Vetter H. Limitations of the reverse transcription-polymerase chain reaction method for the detection of carcinoembryonic antigen-positive tumour cells in peripheral blood. Clin Cancer Res. 1998; 4:2141–2146.
27. Zippelius A, Kufer P, Honold G, *et al.* Limitations of reverse transcriptase-polymerase chain reaction analyses for detection of micrometastatic epithelial cancer cells in bone marrow. J Clin Oncol. 1997; 15:2701.
28. Bostick PJ, Chatterjee S, Chi DD, Huynh KT, Giuliano AE, Cote RJ, Hoon DS. Limitations of specific reverse-transcriptase polymerase chain reaction markers in the detection of metastases in the lymph nodes and blood of breast cancer patients. J Clin Oncol. 1998; 16:2632–2640.
29. Hermanek P, Hutter RVP, Sobin LH, Wittekind Ch. Classification of isolated tumour cells and micrometastasis. Cancer. 1999; 86:2668–2673.
30. Kasper M, Stosiek P, Typlt H, Karsten U. Histological evaluation of three new monoclonal anti-cytokeratin antibodies in normal tissues. Eur J Cancer. 1987; 23: 137–147.
31. Thorban S, Rosenberg R, Busch R, Roder RJ. Epithelial cells in bone marrow of oesophageal cancer patients: a significant prognostic factor by multivariate analysis. Brit J Cancer. 2000; 83:35–39.
32. O'Sullivan GC, Collins JK, O'Brien F, Crowley B, Murphy K, Lee G, Shanahan F. Micrometastases in bone marrow of patients undergoing 'curative' surgery for gastrointestinal cancer. Gastroenterology. 1995; 109:1535–1540.
33. Bonavina L. Early oesophageal cancer: results of a European multicentre survey. Brit J Surg. 1995; 82:98–101.
34. Glickman JN, Torrcs C, Wang HH, Turner JR, Shahsafaei A, Richards WG, Sugarbaker DJ, Odze RD. The prognostic significance of lymph node micrometastasis in patients with esophageal carcinoma. Cancer. 1999; 85:769–778.
35. Woodcock MJ, Eichner R, Nelson WG, Sun TT. Immunolocalization of keratin polypeptides in human epidermis using monoclonal antibodies. J Cell Biol. 1982; 95:580–588.
36. Natsugoe S, Mueller J, Stein HJ, Feith M, Höfler H, Siewert JR. Micrometastasis and tumour cell microinvolvement of lymph nodes from esophageal squamous cell carcinoma: frequency, associated tumour characteristics, and impact on survival. Cancer. 1998; 83:858–866.
37. Matsumoto M, Natsugoe S, Nakashima S, Sakamoto F, Okumura H, Sakita H, Baba M, Takao S, Aikou T. Clinical significance of lymph node micrometastasis of pN0 esophageal squamous cell carcinoma. Cancer Lett. 2000; 153:189–197.
38. Komukai S, Nishimaki T, Watanabe H, Ajioka Y, Suzuki T, Hatakeyama K. Significance of immunohistochemically demonstrated micrometastases to lymph nodes in esophageal cancer with histologically negative nodes. Surgery. 2000; 127:40–46.

39. Latza U, Niedobitek G, Schwarting R, Nekarda N, Stein H. Ber-EP4: new monoclonal antibody which distinguishes epithelia from mesothelia. J Clin Pathol. 1990; 43:213–219.
40. Moll R, Franke WW, Schiller DL, Geiger B, Krepler R. The catalog of human cytokeratins: patterns of expression in normal epithelia, tumours and cultured cells. Cell. 1982; 31:11–24.
41. Bonavina L, Ferrero S, Midolo V, Buffa R, Cesana B, Peracchia A. Lymph node micrometastases in patients with adenocarcinoma of the esophagogastric junction. J Gastrointest Surg. 1999; 3:468–476.
42. Chen Z, Lu X, Huang R. Detection of occult tumour cells in resected lymph nodes of patients with stage I carcinoma and its clinico-pathological significance. Chung Hua Chung Liu Tsa Chih. 1997; 19:69–71.
43. Jung R, Petersen K, Kruger W, Wolf M, Wagener C, Zander A, Neumaier M. Detection of micrometastasis by cytokeratin 20 RT-PCR is limited due to stable background transcription in granulocytes. Brit J Cancer. 1999; 81:870–873.
44. Traweek ST, Liu J, Battifora H. Keratin gene expression in non-epithelial tissues. Detection with polymerase chain reaction. Am J Pathology. 1993; 142:1111.
45. Luketich JD, Kassis ES, Shriver SP, Nguyen NT, Schauer PR, Weigel TL, Yousem SA, Siegfried JM. Detection of micrometastases in histopathologically negative lymph nodes in esophageal cancer. Ann Thorac Surg. 1998; 66:1715–1718.
46. Kassis ES, Nguyen N, Shriver SP, Siegfried JM, Schauer PR, Luketich JD. Detection of occult lymph node metastases in esophageal cancer by minimally invasive staging combined with molecular diagnostic techniques. J Society Laparoendoscopic Surgeons. 1998; 2:331–336.
47. Mori M, Mimori K, Inoue H, Barnard GF, Tsuji K, Nanbara S, Uoe H, Akiyoshi T. Detection of cancer micrometastases in lymph nodes by reverse transcriptase-polymerase chain reaction. Cancer Res. 1995; 55:3417–3420.
48. Kijima F, Natsugoe S, Takao S, Aridome K, Baba M, Yoshifumi M, Eizuru Y, Aikou T. Detection and clinical significance of lymph node micrometastasis determined by reverse transcription-polymerase chain reaction in patients with esophageal carcinoma. Oncology. 2000; 58:38–44.
49. Kano M, Shimada Y, Kaganoi J, Sakurai T, Li Z, Sato F, Watanabe G, Imamura M. Detection of lymph node metastasis of oesophageal cancer by RT-nested PCR for SCC antigen gene mRNA. Brit J Cancer. 2000; 82:429–435.
50. Abe S, Tachibana M, Shiraishi M, Nakamura T. Lymph node metastasis in resectable esophageal cancer. J Thorac Cardiovasc Surg. 1990; 100:287–291.
51. Borgen E, Naume B, Nesland JM, Kvalheim G, Beiske K, Fodstad O, Diel IJ, Solomayer EF, Theocharous P, Coombes RC, Smith BM, Wunder E, Marolleau J-P, Garcia JM, Pantel K. Standardisation of the immunocytochemical detection of cancer cells in bone marrow and blood: I. Establishment of objective criteria for the evaluation of immunostained cells. J Cytotherapy. 1999; 1:377–388.
52. Schütze K, Lahr G. Identification of expressed genes by laser-mediated manipulation of single cells. Nature Biotechnology. 1998; 16:737–742.
53. Dietmaier W, Hartmann A, Wallinger S, Heinmöller E, Kerner T, Endl E, Jauch K-W, Hofstädter F, Ruschoff J. Multiple mutation analyses in single tumour cells with improved whole genome amplification. Am J Pathology. 1999; 154:83–95.
54. Klein CA, Schmidt-Kittler O, Schardt JA, Pantel K, Speicher MR, Riethmueller G. Comparative genomic hybridization, loss of heterozygosity, and DNA sequence analysis of single cells. Proc Natl Acad Sci. 1999; 96:4494–4499.

Chapter 8

CLINICAL RELEVANCE OF TUMOR CELL DISSEMINATION IN COLORECTAL, GASTRIC AND PANCREATIC CARCINOMA

Ilka Vogel, Holger Kalthoff

Molecular Oncology Research Group, Department for General and Thoracic Surgery, University Hospital of Schleswig-Holstein, Campus Kiel, Germany

Abstract
Metastatic spread is a major factor in the prognosis of cancer patients. Early detection and eradication of circulating tumor cells prior to the development of metastases could help to improve the outcome of patients after tumor resection. Disseminated tumor cells have been detected in different compartments of the body using cytological and immunostaining methods and, more recently, using different molecular biological techniques. However, the specificity and the sensitivity of the methods and their prognostic impact are still being debated. This chapter gives an overview over the published studies regarding the prognostic relevance of the detection of disseminated tumor cells in lymph nodes, bone marrow, blood and peritoneal cavity in colorectal, gastric and pancreatic carcinoma patients.

INTRODUCTION

Although the mortality of patients with gastrointestinal carcinoma has been reduced in recent years by (i) early tumor detection, (ii) improved local surgical treatment (1) and (iii) multimodal therapeutic concepts (2), the survival rates of patients are still very unsatisfactory. Haematogeneous dissemination of tumor cells with subsequent development of distant metastases are the main reasons for recurrence in colorectal carcinoma; local recurrence and peritoneal seeding play a more important role in gastric and pancreatic carcinomas.

After curative resection of the primary tumor, the further therapeutic steps are guided by the staging of the primary tumor. The spread in the lymph nodes remains the most important available prognostic indicator so far. But immunohistochemical and molecular-based analyses could demonstrate that micrometastases and often disseminated single tumor cells can be found in patients with histologically negative lymph nodes (Tables 1, 4, 8).

Disseminated tumor cells can also be detected in gastrointestinal carcinoma patients in other compartments like bone marrow, venous blood, the peritoneal

K. Pantel (ed.), Micrometastasis, 139–172.

cavity and other body fluids (urine or pancreatic juice) or in liver biopsies at times conventional staging could not detect residual disease. Therefore, detection of this minimal residual disease will improve the tumor staging and may help to predict prognosis and guide therapeutic decisions (Tables 1–12).

The UICC decided in 2002 that a finding of disseminated tumor cells should not be considered in the TNM-classification. For future evaluation of their prognostic significance it was recommended to document the findings to uniform criteria. As reasons for this restrictive position differences in methodology and non-standardized techniques have been stated (3). However, this criticism also holds true for many so-called conventional staging procedures.

In cases of morphologic examination for isolated tumor cells in lymphatic nodes, the UICC suggest adding the result of these examinations in parentheses, with 'i' as symbol and for non-morphologic examinations the symbol 'mol' (for molecular) accompanied by '+' or '−' for positive or negative results after the N-stage. Disseminated tumor cells in bone marrow, blood, peritoneal washings or other specimens should be added in the same form after the M-stage, including information about the specimen analyzed (3).

The detection of disseminated tumor cells depends on a number of steps, including collection and treatment of the sample, cell separation protocol, chosen antibodies, number of analyzed cells, and evaluation techniques. Although the sensitivity of all different assays varies between 1 tumor cell in 10^6 and 10^7 mononuclear cells (4–9), the detection rate in an individual patient depends on the amount of cells investigated. It has been demonstrated, that multiple samples taken from different sides (for example, bone marrow from the right and left iliac crest) result in higher detection rates compared to one sample (10).

All methods used relay on the recognition of antigens or gene transcripts that are specifically expressed by tumor cells and not by surrounding cells. The great variability in antigenic expression (heterogeneity) between the disseminated tumor cells derived from the primary tumor (11) can, therefore, result in a downregulation or loss of an antigen expression that can be observed in the primary tumor (12–14). For some of the used markers (PSA, mucins) a modulation by hormonal influences has been demonstrated (15, 16).

Irrespective of the methods (immunostaining or RT-PCR), false positive results could also occur due to contamination with skin cells or release of epithelial cells in benign proliferative diseases as far as epithelial markes have been used (6, 17–19; see Tables 1–12); false negative results may occur due to losses of tumor cells during isolation of mononuclear cells (20, 21). PCR-reactions with multiple markers may overcome tumor cell heterogeneity and false positive results. This strategy would also increase sensitivity and specificity of the test.

The enrichment of tumor cells, e.g., by magnetic beads, may improve the results by reducing the background (22–24). However, this procedure is hampered by the heterogeneity in antigen expression of disseminated tumor cells. Further studies will also focus on (semi)-quantitative RT-PCR which allows standardization of the amplification rate and, therefore, false positive results due to extensive amplifications of background gene-expression may be avoided (25).

The studies regarding prognostic relevance performed so far suggest, that the detection of disseminated tumor cells might be useful as criteria to select patients with an unfavorable prognosis who would benefit from adjuvant therapy. A definitive assessment of whether these cells are of prognostic relevance is complicated by the fact that many different methods and markers have been used in multiple detection systems and with different methods of evaluation.

This review summarizes the results of studies of lymph nodes, bone marrow, venous blood, and peritoneal lavage samples taken pre- and intra-operatively and investigated by immunohistochemical and molecular biological techniques in patients with colorectal, gastric and pancreatic carcinomas.

RESULTS OF THE CLINICAL STUDIES AND PROGNOSTIC IMPACT

Various studies have focused on disseminated tumor cells in colorectal, gastric and pancreatic carcinoma in lymph nodes and in bone marrow; few studies have considered tumor cell detection in the peritoneal cavity for these tumors and some other compartments (26–35). The improvements in the application of RT-PCR assays have led to more studies using blood, as this compartment is more readily accessible than bone marrow and allows more frequent analysis.

For a comprehensive overview these studies emphasizing the clinical importance are listed in 12 tables. For each type of carcinoma in the following pages the compartments lymph nodes, bone marrow, venous blood and peritoneal cavity are summarized. The studies regarding detection of disseminated tumor cells in colorectal carcinoma (Tables 1–4) are followed by the studies in patients with gastric (Tables 5–8) and pancreatic carcinoma (Tables 8–12).

COLORECTAL CARCINOMA

Lymph Nodes

Disseminated tumor cells can be detected in a high percentage of the lymph nodes analyzed as negative with conventional pathology. Most of the studies demonstrate, that immunohistochemistry and molecular biological methods are able to increase the detection rates. Depending on the selection of the patients and the marker chosen, the detection rates in N0 lymph nodes range between 2% and 100% (Table 1).

The question whether the detection of disseminated cells in the lymph nodes of patients with colorectal carcinoma is of prognostic impact cannot definitively be answered so far. Immunocytology studies were mainly performed with antibodies directed against cytokeratins. The most often used antibody was CAM 5.2 directed against CK 8, 18, 19. Different results regarding the prognostic impact were

Table 1. Detection of disseminated tumor cells in lymph nodes of patients with colorectal carcinoma

Marker	Antibodies/ Method	Number of Node Negative Patients	Detection Rates (positive patients)	Increase of Detection versus Pathology	Prognostic Relevance	Controls $n=$	Positive Controls	Author
Immunocytochemistry								
CK 8,18,19	CAM 5.2	10	10%	no	**Ø**	Ø	Ø	Makin *et al*. 1989 (44)
CEA+ EMA	anti-CEA+ anti-EMA	28	2%	no	**Ø**	Ø	Ø	Davidson *et al*. 1990 (45)
CEA+ CK	anti-CEA + AE1/AE3	46	26%	yes	− **(u)**	Ø	Ø	Cutait *et al*. 1991 (39)
CK	CAM 5.2	25	48%	yes	**Ø**	Ø	Ø	Haboubi *et al*. 1992 (46)
CK+ TAG72	AE1/AE3 + CC49	50	28% + 76%	yes	+ **(u + m)**	Ø	Ø	Greenson *et al*. 1994 (42)
CK	AE1/AE3	77	25%	yes	− **(u)**	Ø	Ø	Jeffers *et al*. 1994 (47)
CK	CAM 5.2	33	0%	no	**Ø**	6 lym. n.	1%	Nicholson *et al*. 1994 (48)
CK8,18,19	anti-CK 8,18, 19	100	39%	yes	− **(u)**	Ø	Ø	Adell *et al*. 1996 (38)
CK	AE1+ CAM 5.2	16	17.5% of the nodes	yes	**Ø**	Ø	Ø	Cote *et al*. 1996 (49)
CK	AE1/AE3 + BerEP4	32	19%	yes	− **(u)**	Ø	Ø	Broll *et al*. 1997 (50)
CK	CAM 5.2	19	25% of the nodes	yes	+ **hr (u)**	Ø	Ø	Sasaki *et al*.1997 (36)
CK	CAM 5.2	147	32%	yes	− **(u)**	Ø	Ø	Öberg *et al*. 1998 (41)
CK	AE1/AE3+ CAM 5.2	173	59%	yes	**Ø**	Ø	Ø	Hitchcock *et al*. 1999 (51)
CK+ p53	KL-1+ RSP 53	44	KL1: 86%, p53: 44%	yes	− *	Ø	Ø	Nakanishi *et al*. 1999 (40)
CK	CAM 5.2	42	76%	yes	+ **hr (u)**	Ø	Ø	Yasuda *et al*. 2001 (52)

Molecular Biology								
CEA	PCR	1	100%	yes	**Ø**	5	0%	Mori *et al*. 1995 (53)
CEA + CK20	RT-PCR	13	100%	yes	**Ø**	5	0%	Futamura *et al*. 1998 (54)
CEA	RT-PCR	26	54%	yes	+ **(m)**	2	pos.**	Liefers *et al*. 1998 (43)
CEA	RT-PCR	20	40% of the nodes	yes	+ **(u)*****	25	0%	Mori *et al*. 1998 (55)
CEA+ CK 20	RT-PCR	51?	59%(N0/N1) 61% (N0/N1)	yes	**(+) (u)**	?	0%	Rosenberg *et al*. 2000 (56)
CEA+CK20+ CK (IHC)	PCR+ IHC	6	66%	yes	**(+) hr**	Ø	Ø	Miyake *et al*. 2001(57)
CK 19	RT-PCR	15	77% of the nodes	yes	**Ø**	8	85%	Gunn *et al*. 1996 (58)
CK 20		15	24% of the nodes			8	0%	
CK20	PCR	18	22%	yes	**Ø**	5	0%	Dorudi *et al*. 1998 (59)
CK 20	RT-PCR	66	33%	yes	**Ø**	39	2.5%	Merrie *et al*. 1999 (60)
CK 20	RT-PCR	16	88%	yes	**Ø**	22	0%	Weitz *et al*. 1999 (61)
CK 20	RT-PCR	11	54%	yes	**Ø**	41	2%	
K-ras	MASA	11	27%	yes	**Ø**	41	0%	Yun *et al*. 2000 (62)
K-ras, p53	PCR	11	27%	yes	+ **(u)** N0 and N1	Ø	Ø	Sanchez-Cespides *et al*. 1999 (63)
K-ras, CK (IHC)	PCR+ M0821	27	63%	yes	**(+) hr**	Ø	Ø	Clarke *et al*. 2001 (64)
Mucin2	RT-PCR	43	28%	yes	**Ø**	3	0%	Bernini *et al*. 2000 (65)
CD 44	PCR	6	17%	yes	**Ø**	3	0%	Wong *et al*. 1997 (66)
Matrilysin	RT-PCR	60	3% of the nodes	yes	**Ø**	Ø	Ø	Ichikawa *et al*. 1998 (67)
GCC	GCC- PCR	8	25%	yes	**Ø**	Ø	Ø	Waldman *et al*. 1998 (68)
Mammaglobin B	RT-PCR	9	33%	yes	**Ø**	Ø	Ø	Aihara *et al*. 2000 (69)

+: relevant to prognosis, (+): seems relevant to prognosis, but not statistically proven, −: not relevant to prognosis, Ø: not assessed.
m = multivariate analysis, u = univariate analysis, hr = higher recurrence rate.
* case control study, ** (at 20–45cycles), *** multiple carcinoma analysed together.
EMA: epithelial membrane antigen.

observed in these analyses. Some authors found a prognostic relevance for the detection of disseminated tumor cells (36, 37), while other did not (38, 39).

Also the case-controlled study of Nakanishi *et al.* (40) (using the antibodies KL-1 and RSP 53) and the largest study on 147 patients performed by Öberg *et al.* (41) (using the antibody CAM 5.2) could not demonstrate an influence of the detection of disseminated tumor cells on survival. The only multivariate analyses were performed by Greenson *et al.* 1994 (IHC: AE1/AE3 and CC49)(42) and by Liefers *et al.* 1998 (CEA-RT-PCR) (43). Both demonstrate the prognostic influence of the detection of disseminated cells in lymph nodes of colorectal carcinoma patients. An independent confirmation by multivariate analyses of larger series of patients is needed, but the prognostic impact of the detection of disseminated tumor cells in lymph nodes of patients with colorectal carcinoma seems to be quite obvious.

Bone Marrow

Immunohistochemical analyses of bone marrow samples of patients with colorectal carcinoma were performed initially by Schlimok *et al.* (70) with the monoclonal antibody CK2 which specifically reacts with cytokeratin 18 (CK18). Further studies with the same antibody showed detection rates in bone marrow between 16% and 32%. Other studies using combinations of antibodies found disseminated cells in bone marrow in up to 74% of cases, whereas PCR-mediated tests yielded positive results in 24% to 89% of the patients (Table 2). Specificity was evaluated in all studies by analyzing samples from patients without evidence of any carcinoma or from healthy subjects. Most of the studies had a false positive rate of below 10%. This will not allow the introduction of such analyses as a routine procedure.

Using multivariate analysis, Lindemann (71) showed that the detection of disseminated tumor cells in the bone marrow with the monoclonal antibody CK2 is an independent prognostic factor for survival. Leinung *et al.* (72) also found a significant influence by using the pan-specific cytokeratin antibody A45-B/B3 which detects a common epitope on a variety of cytokeratin types, including CK8,18, and 19.

Other authors combined different antibodies directed against cytokeratins, and/or tumor-associated antigens, but no multivariate analyses were performed in any of these studies to demonstrate prognostic relevance. Since tumor-associated antigens or epithelia-specific antigens can be illegitimately expressed in haematopoietic cells (73, 74), and as pseudogenes may cause PCR products of identical size (18), the RT-PCR assays resulted in a high number of false positive signals (Table 2). So far, CK20 seems to be the best marker, although some false positive results have been observed here as well (19, 75). Our analyses of 226 curatively resected patients have shown for the first time that the detection of disseminated tumor cells in bone marrow is a prognostic factor for overall survival in patients with colorectal carcinoma (76), but this needs to be confirmed by a even larger series and longer follow-up time.

Table 2. Detection of disseminated tumor cells in bone marrow of patients with colorectal carcinoma

Marker/ Antibodies	Number of Patients	Detection Rates	Stage Dependent Increase of Detection	Prognostic Relevance	Controls *n* =	Positive Controls	Author
Immunocytochemistry							
CK 18 (Mab: CK2)	57	12/ 57 (21%)	+	**Ø**	75	0%	Schlimok *et al.* 1987 (70)
CK 18 (Mab: CK2)	82	22/82 (27%)	+	**Ø**	75	0%	Schneider *et al.* 1989 (77)
CK 18 (Mab: CK2)	156	42/156 (27%)	+	+ **(u)**	102	0%	Schlimok *et al.*1990 (78)
CK 18 (Mab: CK2)	88	2/88 (32%)	+	+ **(u + m)**	102	0%	Lindemann *et al.* 1992 (71)
CK 18 (Mab: CK2)	57	9/57 (16%)	+	**Ø**	75	5.5%	Pantel *et al.* 1994 (10)
CK 18 (FACS)	48	11/48 (23%)	+	**Ø**	63	1.5%	O'Sullivan *et al.* 1997 (135)
CEA, Ca 19-9, CD 54-0, Ra 96, 17-1-A, KL-1	58	17/58 (29%)	+	**Ø**	25	0%	Juhl *et al.* 1994 (6)
KL-1, CK2, anti-CEA, 17-1-A	34	20/27 (74%)	+	**Ø**	Ø	Ø	Broll *et al.* 1996 (80)
A33, AE1, CK 18, Cam 5.2	80	resected 9% non-res. 34%	**Ø**	− **(u)**	20	0%	Cohen *et al.* 1998 (81)
CEA, Ca 19-9, CD 54-0, Ra 96, 17-1-A, KL-1	105	35/1205 (33%)	+	− **(u)**	45	4%	Schott *et al.* 1998 (82)
CK 20 + FISH	18	16/18 (89%)	**Ø**	**Ø**	12	58%	Litle *et al.* 1997 (83)
CK (A45-B/B3)	145	36/145 (24%)	**Ø**	+ **(u + m)**	51	0%	Leinung *et al.* 2000 (72)
Molecular Biology							
CEA	6	4/6 (66%)	**Ø**	**Ø**	56	0%	Gerhard *et al.* 1994 (75)
CK19+	15	6 /15 (40%)	**Ø**	**Ø**	4	41%	Gunn *et al.* 1996 (58)
CK20	15	0/15 (0%)	**Ø**	**Ø**	4	0%	
CK 20	57	20/57 (35%)	**Ø**	+ **(dis. free) (u)**	16	6%	Soeth *et al.* 1996 (19)
CK 20	65	20/65 (31%)	+	+ **(u)**	22	9%	Soeth *et al.* 1997 (84)
CK 20	14	3/14 (21%)	**Ø**	**Ø**	Ø	Ø	Weitz *et al.* 1999 (61)
CK 20	30	8/30 (27%)	**Ø**	**Ø**	30	0%	Weitz *et al.* 2000 (85)
CK 20	226	71/226 (31%)	+	+ **(u)**	22	9%	Vogel *et al.* 2000 (76)

+: relevant to prognosis, (+): seems relevant to prognosis, but not statistically proven, −: not relevant to prognosis, Ø: not assessed.
m = multivariate analysis, u = univariate analysis, hr = higher recurrence rate.

Table 3. Detection of disseminated tumor cells in blood of patients with colorectal carcinoma

Marker/ Antibodies	Number of Patients	Detection Rates	Stage Dependent Increase of Detection	Prognostic Relevance	Controls $n =$	Positive Controls	Author
Molecular Biology							
K-ras	27	9/27 (33%)	+	**+ (u) dis. free**	Ø	Ø	Hardingham *et al*. 1995 (86)
p53	41	17/41 (42%)	**Ø**	**Ø**	10	0%	Khan *et al*. 2000 (88)
CEA	31	26/31 Stage IV (84%)	**Ø**	**Ø**	22	0%	Jonas *et al*. 1996 (89)
CEA	20	7/20 (35%)	**Ø**	**Ø**	22	0%	Mori *et al*. 1996 (90)
CEA	95	39/95 (41%)	+	**Ø**	11 healthy 9 inflamm.	0% 55%	Castells *et al*. 1998 (91)
CEA	0	Ø	**Ø**	**Ø**	24	33%	Ko *et al*. 1998 (92)
CEA	27	10/27 (38%)	**Ø**	**Ø**	22%	0%	Mori *et al*. 1998 (55)
CEA	24	9/24 (38%)	**Ø**	**Ø**	9	0%	Noh *et al*. 1999 (93)
CEA	53	18/53 (34%)	+	**+ (u)**	32	0%	Taniguchi *et al*. 2000 (94)
CEA	69	27/69 (34%)	+	**Ø**	8	25%	Piva *et al*. 2000 (95)
CEA	51	34/51 (67%)	+	**Ø**	78	2.5%	Guadagni *et al*. 2001 (96)
CEA	95 68 R0	39/95 (41%) 26/68 (38%)	+	**− (u + m)**	Ø	Ø	Bessa *et al*. 2001 (97)
CD44	24	4/24 (17%)	**Ø**	**Ø**	8	0%	Wong *et al*. 1997 (66)
CK19,20,8	23	12/23 (52%)	**Ø**	**Ø**	42	0%	Denis *et al*. 1997 (22)
CK19	27	7/27 (26%)	**Ø**	**Ø**	21	30%	Bustin *et al*. 1999 (26)
CK20	27	27/27 (100%)			21	100%	
GCC	27	20 /27 (74%)			21	5%	
CK19	10	2/10 (20%)	**Ø**	**Ø**	Ø	Ø	Masson *et al*. 2000 (98)
CD44v6	10	3/10 (30%)			6	100%	
CK19, CK20, MUC1, MUC2	94	19/64 (all markers) (20%)	+	**+ (u + m) (all markers)**	20 healthy 30 adenom 34 inflam.	0% 10% 12%	Hardingham *et al*. 2000 (87)
CK8, CK19,	0	Ø	**Ø**	**Ø**	9 15	89% 40%	Burchill *et al*. 1995 (99)

CK20	52	9/52 (17%)	+	+ **(u)**	58	3%	Soeth *et al*. 1997 (84)
CK20	35	0/35 (0%)	**Ø**	**Ø**	19	0%	Nakamori *et al*. 1997 (100)
CK20	8	6/8 (75%)	**Ø**	**Ø**	6	0%	Funaki *et al*. 1997 (101)
CK20	28	18/28 (55%)	+	**(+) rec.**	11	0%	Funaki *et al*. 1998 (102)
CK20	25	12/25 (48%)	−	− **(u)**	12	8%	Wyld *et al*. 1998 (103)
CK20	65	24/58 (46%)	+	**Ø**	12	0%	Weitz *et al*. 1998 (104)
		6/8 liver res. (86%)					
CK20	5	3/5 (60%)	**Ø**	**Ø**	29	72%	Champelovier *et al*. 1999 (105)
CK20	35	11/35 (31%)	+	**Ø**	22	0%	Chausovsky *et al*. 1999 (106)
CK20	0	Ø	**Ø**	**Ø**	33	0%	Jung *et al*. 1999 (73)
CK20+	100	34/100 (34%)	**Ø**	**Ø**	70	1%	Wharton *et al*. 1999 (107)
CEA		48/100 (48%)			70	3%	
		combined (78%)			70	4.2%	
CK20	16	2/16 (12.5%)	**Ø**	**Ø**	12	0%	Weitz *et al*. 1999 (61)
CK20	8	6/8 (75%)	**Ø**	**Ø**	3	0%	Funaki *et al*. 2000 (108)
CK20 + CEA	55	44/55 (80%)	**Ø**	**Ø**	85	5%	Patel *et al*. 2000 (109)
CK20	243	82/243 (38%)	+	+ **(u)**	58	3%	Vogel *et al*. 2000 (76)
CK20	41	26/41 (63%)	**Ø**	**Ø**	31	0%	Weitz *et al*. 2000 (85)
CK20 + CEA	52	8/52 combined (15%)	+	− **(u)**	20	0%	Yamaguchi *et al*. 2000 (110)
CK20 + CEA	33	28/33 combined (85%)	**Ø**	**Ø**	70	1.4%	Mathur *et al*. 2001 (111)
					70	2.8%	

+: relevant to prognosis, (+): seems relevant to prognosis, but not statistically proven, −: not relevant to prognosis, Ø: not assessed.
m = multivariate analysis, u = univariate analysis.
dis. free = disease-free survival, rec. = tumor recurrence, inflamm. = inflammatory diseases , hr = higher recurrence rate.

Blood

Due to the increased sensitivity compared to immunohistochemical analyses, many molecular biological studies have presented the detection of disseminated tumor cell blood of patients with colorectal carcinoma (Table 3). As marker genes cytokeratins were mainly used as epithelial markers in the mesenchymal compartments. A problem of these markers is the high rate of false positive results if the analyses are performed from whole blood. Jung *et al.* (73) demonstrated, that granulocytes express CK20, and false positive signals caused by other blood cells are discussed. Therefore, the isolation of mononuclear cells by Ficoll or other techniques is necessary.

One other possibility is the combination of different markers as performed by Hardingham *et al.* (87). This is so far the only study demonstrating a prognostic relevance for the detection of disseminated tumor cells in venous blood in colorectal carcinoma patients by multivariate analysis. In our own large series of 243 curatively resected patients, we could demonstrate a prognostic influence for the detection by CK20 RT-PCR in univariate analysis so far (76).

Peritoneal Lavage

Tumor cell dissemination in the abdominal cavity in colorectal carcinoma occurs mostly in very late tumor stages in colorectal carcinoma, and compared to pancreatic and gastric carcinoma, only a few studies analyzed the question of disseminated tumor cells in the peritoneal cavity of colorectal carcinoma patients. To date, none of the studies analyzing peritoneal washings has demonstrated, that the detection of disseminated tumor cells in patients with colorectal carcinoma is of independent prognostic importance (Table 4).

GASTRIC CARCINOMA

Lymph Nodes

In the lymph nodes of patients with gastric carcinoma disseminated tumor cells can be detected in over 25% of the pathologically negative lymph nodes. In most of the studies anti-cytokeratin antibodies have been used. But even by the use of the same antibody for cytokeratins (CAM5.2), the detection rate differs from 17% to 90%. The prognostic impact was demonstrated in univariate analysis in some studies (115–117), whereas in other studies (118–121) it was not. Only one group (published in 2 papers) performed a multivariate analysis (122, 123), and demonstrated a prognostic influence for those patients who were staged N0 by conventional pathology. This group used a different anti-cytokeratin antibody (AE1/AE3); no other authors have confirmed these results so far.

Molecular biological analyses were performed only in a small series (Table 5) and will require further efforts.

Table 4. Detection of disseminated tumor cells in peritoneal lavage of patients with colorectal carcinoma

Marker/ Antibodies	Number of Patients	Detection Rates	Stage Dependent Increase of Detection	Prognostic Relevance	Controls *n* =	Positive Controls	Author
Immunocytochemistry							
CEA L11/285/14, HMGFG 1 and 2	30	3/30 (13%)	**Ø**	**Ø**	Ø	Ø	Ambrose *et al.* 1995 (112)
CEA, Ca 19-9, CD 54-0, Ra 96, 17-1-A	60	16/60 (27%)	+	**Ø**	33	0%	Juhl *et al.* 1994 (113)
KL-1, CK 2,anti-CEA, 17-1-A	30	20/30 (67%)		**Ø**	Ø	Ø	Broll *et al.* 1996 (80)
CEA, Ca 19-9, CD 54-0, Ra 96, 17-1-A	109	34/109 (31%)	+	+ **(u)**	45	6%	Schott *et al.* 1998 (82)
CEA	49	8/49 (16%)	+	+ **(u)***	13	0%	Broll *et al.* 2001 (114)
Molecular Biology							
CEA PCR	49	32/49 (65%)	+	+ **(u)***	13	38%	Broll *et al.* 2001 (114)

+: relevant to prognosis, (+): seems relevant to prognosis, but not statistically proven, −: not relevant to prognosis, Ø: not assessed.
m = multivariate analysis, u = univariate analysis, hr = higher recurrence rate.
* R0–R2, overall gastric, colorectal and pancreatic carcinoma.

Table 5. Detection of disseminated tumor cells in lymph nodes of patients with gastric carcinoma

Marker	Antibodies/ Method	Number of Node Negative Patients	Detection Rates (positive patients)	Increase of Detection versus Pathology	Prognostic Relevance	Controls $n =$	Positive Controls	Author
Immunocytochemistry								
CK	AE1/AE3/ BerEP4	100	90%	yes	**+ (u + m)**	Ø	Ø	Siewert *et al.* 1996 (123)
CK+		109	8.8% of the nodes	yes	**+ (u)**	Ø	Ø	Ishida *et al.* 1997 (124)
CEA			3% of the nodes					
CK	AE1/AE3	113	90%	yes	**+ (u + m)**	Ø	Ø	Kestlmeier *et al.* 1997
(122)								
CK	AE1/AE3	67	21%	yes	**+ (u)**	Ø	Ø	Nakajo *et al.* 2001 (125)
CK 18	Anti CK 18	40	7.5%	yes	**− (u)**	Ø	Ø	Stachura *et al.* 1998 (121)
CK	CAM 5.2	34	23.5%	yes	**+ (u)**	Ø	Ø	Maehara *et al.* 1996 (117)
CK	CAM 5.2	79	25%	yes	**(+) (u)**	Ø	Ø	Cai *et al.* 2000 (126)
CK	CAM 5.2	25	36%	yes	**+ (u)**	Ø	Ø	Harrison *et al.* 2000 (115)
CK	CAM 5.2	91	68%	yes	**Ø**	Ø	Ø	Ikeguchi *et al.* 2000 (116)
CK	CAM 5.2	139	17%	yes	**− (u)**	Ø	Ø	Saragoni *et al.* 2000 (120)
CK+	CAM 5.2	160	27.5%	yes	**(+) hr**	Ø	Ø	Ikeguchi *et al.* 2001 (181)
Cathepsin D	CD							
CK		107	35.5%	yes	**− (u)**	Ø	Ø	Fukagawa *et al.* 2001 (118)
CK		139	17%	yes	**− (u)**	Ø	Ø	Morgagni *et al.* 2001 (119)
Molecular Biology								
CEA	RT-PCR	4	50%	yes	**Ø**	5	0%	Mori *et al.* 1995 (53)
CK 19	RT-PCR	12	15%	yes	**Ø**	20 lym.n	0%	Noguchi *et al.* 1996 (127)
CEA	RT-PCR	31	40% of the nodes	yes	**+ (u)***	25	0%	Mori *et al.* 1998 (55)
Mammaglobin B	RT-PCR	32 nodes	22%	yes	**Ø**	Ø	Ø	Aihara *et al.* 2000 (69)
CEA/CK 20/ MAGE3	RT-PCR	28	36%	yes	**(+) hr**	16	0%	Okada *et al.* 2001 (129)

+: relevant to prognosis, (+): seems relevant to prognosis, but not statistically proven, −: not relevant to prognosis, Ø: not assessed.
m = multivariate, u = univariate analysis, hr = higher recurrence rate.
* Multiple carcinomas analyzed together.

Bone Marrow

Detection rates in the bone marrow ranged between 25% and 82% by immunocytochemical analysis (Table 6). Overall, the detection rate seems to be slightly higher than in colorectal carcinoma.

Only one study published by Jauch (130) included a multivariate analysis demonstrating that the presence of three or more cells in the bone marrow was of prognostic significance for disease-free survival for patients with T1/2 tumors only. Heiss *et al.* (131) showed that tumor cell dissemination in bone marrow was an additional prognostic factor in early tumor stages (UICC I/II) and lymph-node negative (N0) patients combined with a predictive factor given by the expression of the urokinase plasminogen activator (uPA)-receptor.

Molecular biological analyses have been performed with CEA, CK19 and CK20 as markers (Table 6). Up to now only the analyses of our own group, including 49 bone marrow samples and 18 venous blood samples, had demonstrated in univariate analyses a significant difference in overall survival for patients with tumor cells in bone marrow and blood (84). It is noticeable that the detection rate in bone marrow was low compared to immunocytochemical studies, although advanced stages were included. The most likely explanation for this is, that CK20 is not expressed in all gastric carcinomas.

Blood

Disseminated tumor cells in the blood of patients with gastric carcinoma have been detected only by molecular biological methods (Table 7). As markers CEA, CK19 and CK20 (132, 133) have been used. Only one study analyzed more than 50 patients with gastric carcinoma, therefore statements regarding the prognostic impact are not yet justified.

Peritoneal Lavage

Detection rates between 18% and 100% were observed in the peritoneal cavity of patients with gastric carcinoma (Table 8). This rather high detection rate might be explained by the higher rate of peritoneal carcinosis at the time of primary operation in gastric carcinoma compared to colorectal cancer. Most studies revealed a prognostic impact on survival; in four studies this was found to be an independent prognostic factor.

In gastric cancer patients detection of disseminated tumor cells without macroscopically visible carcinosis seems to lead to peritoneal carcinosis in the near future. The detection rates in gastric cancer also depend on patient selection and the used markers.

Table 6. Detection of disseminated tumor cells in bone marrow of patients with gastric carcinoma

Marker/ Antibodies	Number of Patients	Detection Rates	Stage Dependent Increase of Detection	Prognostic Relevance	Controls $n =$	Positive Controls	Author
Immunocytochemistry							
CK18 (mab:CK2)	97	34/97 (35%)	+	+ **(u)**	75	0%	Schlimok *et al.* 1991 (134)
CK18 + uPA-R	78	47/78 (60%)	**Ø**	− **(u)**	Ø	Ø	Heiss *et al.* 1995 (131)
CK18 (FACS)	57	16/57 (28%)	**Ø**	**Ø**	Ø	Ø	O'Sullivan *et al.* 1995 (79)
CK18 (mab:CK2)	102	45/102 (44%)	**Ø**	**Ø**	Ø	Ø	Funke *et al.* 1996 (136)
CK18 (mab:CK2)	180	95/180 (53%)	+	+ **(u, m (T1/2 N0))**	64	0%	Jauch *et al.* 1996 (130)
CK18 (mab:CK2)	46	15/46 (33%)	**Ø**	**Ø**	Ø	Ø	Maehara *et al.* 1996 (117)
CK18 (uPA-R)	78	47/78 (60%)	**Ø**	(+) **hr**	?	0%	Allgayer *et al.* 1997 (137)
CK18 (FACS)	15	5/15 (33%)	**Ø**	**Ø**	63	1.5%	O'Sullivan *et al.* 1997 (135)
CK18 (mab:CK2)	53	27/53 (51%)	+	− **(u)**	Ø	Ø	Kerner *et al.* 1998 (138)
CK	88	58/88 (66%)	+	**Ø**	Ø	Ø	Liu *et al.* 1995 (139)
CEA, Ca 19-9, CD 54-0, Ra 96, 17-1-A KL-1	36	9/36 (25%)	+	**Ø**	25	0%	Juhl *et al.* 1994 (113)
KL-1, CK2, anti-CEA, 17-1-A	17	14/17 (82%)	+	**Ø**	Ø	Ø	Broll *et al.* 1996 (80)
CEA, Ca 19-9, CD 54-0, Ra 96, 17-1-A, KL-1	60	30/60 (48%)	+	− **(u)**	45	4%	Schott *et al.* 1998 (82)
Molecular Biology							
CEA	2	2/2 (100%)	**Ø**	**Ø**	56	0%	Gerhard *et al.* 1994 (75)
CK20	49	11/49 (22%)	+	+ **(u)**	22	9%	Soeth *et al.* 1997 (84)

+: relevant to prognosis, (+): seems relevant to prognosis, but not statistically proven, −: not relevant to prognosis, Ø: not assessed.
m = multivariate analysis, u = univariate analysis, hr = higher recurrence rate.

Table 7. Detection of disseminated tumor cells in blood of patients with gastric carcinoma

Marker/ Antibodies	Number of Patients	Detection Rates	Stage Dependent Increase of Detection	Prognostic Relevance	Controls *n*=	Positive Controls	Author
Immunocytochemistry Molecular Biology							
CEA	9	2/9 (22%)	**Ø**	**Ø**	13	0%	Funaki *et al.* 1996 (180)
CEA	20	7/20 (35%)	**Ø**	**Ø**	22	0%	Mori *et al.* 1996 (90)
CEA	62	12/62 (19%)	**Ø**	**Ø**	22	0%	Mori *et al.* 1998 (55)
CEA	41	gastroint. tumcrs 8/22 R0 (22%) 4/5 R2 (80%)	+	**Ø**	Ø	Ø	Nishida *et al.* 2000 (167)
CEA	30	11/30 (37%)	+	**Ø**	8	25%	Piva *et al.* 2000 (95)
CEA	57	21/57 (37%)	+	(+) **hr**	30	0%	Miyazono *et al.* 2001 (142)
CK19	40	2/40 (5%)	**Ø**	**Ø**	50	0% (2x pos.) 16% (1x pos.)	Aihara *et al.* 1997 (128)
CK20	30	3/30 (17%)	+	+ **(u)**	58	3%	Soeth *et al.* 1997 (84)
CK20	18	12/18 met. pat. (67%)	**Ø**	**Ø**	22	0%	Chausovsky *et al.* 1999 (106)

+: relevant to prognosis, (+): seems relevant to prognosis, but not statistically proven, −: not relevant to prognosis, Ø: not assessed.
m = multivariate analysis, u = univariate analysis, hr = higher recurrence rate.

Table 8. Detection of disseminated tumor cells in peritoneal lavage of patients with gastric carcinoma

Marker/ Antibodies	Number of Patients	Detection Rates	Stage Dependent Increase of Detection	Prognostic Relevance	Controls *n* =	Positive Controls	Author
Immunocytochemistry							
CK (B72.3)	18	6/18 (33%)	**Ø**	**Ø**	?	0%	Murphy *et al.* 1993 (143)
CEA, Ca 19-9, CD 54-0, Ra 96, 17-1-A, KL-1	44	19/44 (43%)	+	**Ø**	33	0%	Juhl *et al.* 1994 (113)
Be-EP4, B72.3, CEA, 17-1-A	18	13/18 (72%)	−	**Ø**	Ø	Ø	Broll *et al.* 1996 (80)
B72.3, AR3, BD5	144	50/144 (35%)	+	+ **(u)**	Ø	Ø	Benevelo *et al.* 1998 (144)
CEA, Ca 19-9, CD 54-0, Ra 96, 17-1-A	62	33/62 (53%)	+	+ **(u)**	45	6%	Schott *et al.* 1998 (82)
CEA, Ca 19-9, STN, SLX	51	16/51 (32%)	**Ø**	**Ø**	Ø	Ø	Imada *et al.* 1999 (145)
CK (Ber-Ep4)	118	23/118 (20%)	+	+ **(u + m))**	Ø	Ø	Nekarda *et al.* 1999 (146)
CEA (Elisa)	56	10/56 (18%)	+	+ **(u + m)**	20	0%	Abe *et al.* 2001 (147)
CEA	17	5/17 (29%)	+	+ **(u)***	13	0%	Broll *et al.* 2001 (114)
Matrix Metalloproteinase 7	152	27/152 (18%)	+	+ **(u + m)**	26	0%	Yonemura *et al.* 2001 (37)
Molecular Biology							
CEA PCR + Cytology	148	41/148 (28%)	+	+ **(u)**	Ø	Ø	Kodera *et al.* 1998 (148)
CEA PCR	17	8/17 (47%)	−	+ **(u)***	13	38%	Broll *et al.* 2001 (114)
CEA light cycler PCR	241	88% sensitivity	+	(+)	?	12%	Nakanishi *et al.* 2001 (149)
Trypsinogen PCR+IHC	8	4/8 (50%)	+	**Ø**	Ø	Ø	Fujimura *et al.* 1998 (150)
E-cadherin PCR + cytology	52	52/52 (100%) 8/52 (15.3%)	**Ø**	**Ø**	5	PCR:100%	Schuhmacher *et al.* 1999 (151)
Telomerase PCR	20	10/20 (50%) IHC: 9/20 (45%)	**Ø**	**Ø**	5	0%	Mori *et al.* 2000 (152)
Matrix Metallo-proteinase 7-PCR	152	28/152 (18%)	+	+ **(u + m)**	26	0%	Yonemura *et al.* 2001 (37)

+: relevant to prognosis, (+): seems relevant to prognosis, but not statistically proven, −: not relevant to prognosis, Ø: not assessed.
m = multivariate analysis, u = univariate analysis, hr = higher recurrence rate.
* R0–R2, overall gastric, colorectal and pancreatic carcinoma.

PANCREATIC CARCINOMA

Still fewer studies have considered patients with pancreatic carcinoma. This may be a reflection of the overall poor prognosis for these patients and the lower incidence of the disease compared to colorectal or gastric carcinoma.

Lymph Nodes

The immunohistochemical detection of disseminated tumor cells in lymph nodes from pancreatic carcinoma patients was shown to be of prognostic significance in a multivariate analysis by Hosch *et al.* (153), but only 18 patients were included in this study (Table 9).

The high rate of ki-ras mutations in pancreatic carcinoma represents a hallmark in this disease. The search for disseminated tumor cells on a molecular biological basis focused on this marker. But only one of four studies could demonstrate a prognostic impact in univariate analysis so far (154).

Bone Marrow

Immunohistochemical analyses of bone marrow samples have been performed with cocktails of antibodies, including Ca 19-9 as a typical tumor-associated antigen. In view of the higher number of advanced-stage patients in the respective series, detection rates of disseminated cells of almost 40% to 60% have been found (Table 10). In univariate analysis most of the studies demonstrated a reduced survival rate in patients with detection of tumor cells in bone marrow. Our own series of 80 patients demonstrated a statistical trend but not a significant difference in survival (160).

Molecular biological analyses have been performed in only a small number of cases. Obviously, these markers will need evaluation in a larger series.

Blood

A study of detection of disseminated tumor cells in blood of patients with pancreatic carcinoma based on immunohistochemistry was performed by Z'graggen *et al.* (164) demonstrating no influence on survival in uni- and multivariate analyses (Table 11).

The ten studies performed with molecular biological techniques so far reported possible markers for the detection of disseminated tumor cells. However, the small numbers and in some studies low detection rates (4%, Aihara *et al.* (128); 9%, Soeth *et al.* (84)) of analyzed patients did not allow conclusions regarding the prognostic impact on survival.

Table 9. Detection of disseminated tumor cells in lymph nodes of patients with pancreatic carcinoma

Marker	Antibodies/ Method	Number of Node Negative Patients	Detection Rate (positive patients)	Increase of Detection versus Pathology	Prognostic Relevance	Controls $n =$	Positive Controls	Author
Immunocytochemistry								
CK	Ber-EP4	18	13/18 (72.2%)	yes	**+ (m)**	Ø	Ø	Hosch *et al.* 1997 (153)
Ca19-9	Anti-Ca19-9	15	15/15 (100%)	yes	**Ø**	11	64%	Ridwelski *et al.* 2001 (155)
CK	AE1/AE3	15	15/15 (100%)			11	0%	
Molecular Biology								
K-ras	RT-PCR	12	10/12 (83%)	yes	**+ (u)**	Ø	Ø	Tamagawa *et al.* 1997 (154)
K-ras	RT-PCR	15	8/13 (61.5%)	yes	**Ø**	Ø	Ø	Ando *et al.* 1997 (156)
K-ras	RT-PCR	22	16/22 (73%)	yes	**Ø**	5	0%	Demeure *et al.* 1998 (157)
K-ras	RT-PCR	25	17/25 (68%)	yes	**Ø** **+ with adjuv. trea.**	5	0%	Demeure *et al.* 1998 (158)
K-ras+ CK-IHC	RT-PCR+ AE1/AE3	30	19/30 (47%) PCR 19/30 (63%) IHC	yes yes	**− (u)**	Ø	Ø	Brown *et al.* 2001 (159)

+: relevant to prognosis, (+): seems relevant to prognosis, but not statistically proven, −: not relevant to prognosis, Ø: not assessed.
m = multivariate analysis, u = univariate analysis, hr = higher recurrence rate.

Table 10. Detection of disseminated tumor cells in bone marrow of patients with pancreatic carcinoma

Marker/ Antibodies	Number of Patients	Detection Rates	Stage Dependent Increase of Detection	Prognostic Relevance	Controls *n* =	Positive Controls	Author
Immunocytochemistry							
CEA, Ca 19-9, CD 54-0, Ra 96, 17-1-A ,KL-1	32	15/26 (58%)	+	**Ø**	25	0	Juhl *et al.* 1994 (113)
CK 2, KL-1, A45/B/B3	42	24/42 (57%)	**Ø**	–	25	0	Thorban *et al.* 1996 (161)
CK 2, KL-1, A45/B/B3	48	25/48 (52%)	+	+ **(u)**	25	0	Thorban *et al.* 1999 (162)
CK 2, KL-1, A45/B/B3	48	14/31 resected (48%) 10/18 not res. (59%)	+	+ **(u)**	33	0	Roder *et al.* 1999 (163)
CEA, Ca 19-9, CD 54-0, Ra 96, 17-1-A , KL-1	80	27/71 (38%)	+	**(+) (u)**	45	4%	Vogel *et al.* 1999 (160)
AE1/AE3	54	13/54 (24%)	–	– **(u + m)**	66	0%	Z'graggen *et al.* 2001 (164)
Molecular Biology							
CEA	3	2/3 (66%)	**Ø**	**Ø**	56	0	Gerhard *et al.* 1994 (75)
CK 20	11	4/11 (36%)	**Ø**	**Ø**	16	6%	Soeth *et al.* 1996 (19)
CK 20	27	5/27 (19%)	+	**Ø**	22	9%	Soeth *et al.* 1997 (84)

+: relevant to prognosis, (+): seems relevant to prognosis, but not statistically proven, –: not relevant to prognosis, Ø: not assessed.
m = multivariate analysis, u = univariate analysis, hr = higher recurrence rate.

Table 11. Detection of disseminated tumor cells in blood of patients with pancreatic carcinoma

Marker/ Antibodies	Number of Patients	Detection Rates	Stage Dependent Increase of Detection	Prognostic Relevance	Controls *n* =	Positive Controls	Author
Immunocytochemistry							
AE1/AE3	105	27/105 (26%) 3/32 R0 (9%)	+	**− (u + m)**	66	1.5%	Z'graggen *et al.* 2001 (164)
Molecular Biology							
K-ras	6	2/6 (33%)	**Ø**	**Ø**	2	0%	Tada *et al.* 1993 (165)
K-ras	10	0/10 Preop (0%) 5/10 Intraop (50%)	**Ø**	**Ø**	Ø	Ø	Nomoto *et al.*1996 (166)
CEA	9	3/9 (33%)	**Ø**	**Ø**	13	0%	Funaki *et al.* 1996 (180)
CEA	21	13/21 (62%)	+	**Ø**	15	0%	Miyazono *et al.* 1999 (142)
CEA	27	1/27 (41%)	−	**Ø**	8	25%	Piva *et al.* 2000 (95)
CK19	49	2/49 (4%)	+	**Ø**	12	0%	Aihara *et al.* 1997 (128)
CK20	22	2/22 (9%)	+	**Ø**	58	3.5%	Soeth *et al.* 1997 (84)
CK20	28	22/28 Stage IV (78%)	**Ø**	**Ø**	22	0%	Chausovsky *et al.* 1999 (106)
Chytrypsinogen	10	7/10 (70%)	+	**Ø**	10	0%	Kuroki *et al.* 1999 (168)
MET, GalNacT, β-hCG	33	17/17 Stage IV (100%) 8/16 (MET + Gal) 7/16 (β-HCG)	+	**Ø**	22	0%	Bilchik *et al.* 2000 (169)

+: relevant to prognosis, (+): seems relevant to prognosis, but not statistically proven, −: not relevant to prognosis, Ø: not assessed.
m = multivariate analysis, u = univariate analysis, hr = higher recurrence rate.

Table 12. Detection of disseminated tumor cells in peritoneal lavage of patients with pancreatic carcinoma

Marker/ Antibodies	Number of Patients	Detection Rates	Stage Dependent Increase of Detection	Prognostic Relevance	Controls *n* =	Positive Controls	Author
Immunocytochemistry							
CEA, Ca 19-9, CD 54-0, Ra 96, 17-1-A	31	18/31 (58%)	+	**Ø**	33	0	Juhl *et al*. 1994 (6)
Ca 19-9, CEA	20	4/20 (20%)	**Ø**	**Ø**	5	0	Nomoto *et al*. 1997 (172)
CEA, Ca 19-9, B72.3, Leu-M1	137	32/137 (23%)	**Ø**	**+ (u)**	Ø	Ø	Makary *et al*. 1998 (170)
Ca 19-9, CEA	74	14/66 (22%)	**Ø**	**− (u)**	Ø	Ø	Nakao *et al*. 1999 (171)
CEA, Ca 19-9, CD 54-0, Ra 96, 17-1-A	80	24/62 (39%)	+	**+ (u)**	45	6%	Vogel *et al*. 1999 (160)
CEA	9	4/9 (44%)	+	**+ (u + m)***	13	0	Broll *et al*. 2001 (114)
Molecular Biology							
K-ras	24	2/4 (8%) cytology 3/24 (12%)	**Ø**	**Ø**	14	0	Rall *et al*. 1995 (173)
K-ras	20	2/20 (10%)	+	**Ø**	5	0	Inoue *et al*. 1995 (174) Nomoto *et al*. 1997 (172)
CEA	9	7/9 (78%)	+	**− (u + m)***	13	38%	Broll *et al*. 2001 (114)

+: relevant to prognosis, (+): seems relevant to prognosis, but not statistically proven, −: not relevant to prognosis, Ø: not assessed.
m = multivariate analysis, u = univariate analysis, hr = higher recurrence rate.
* R0–R2, overall gastric, colorectal and pancreatic carcinoma.

Peritoneal Lavage

Many cytological studies have been performed in patients with pancreatic carcinoma, but only few using immunohistochemical or molecular biological methods (Table 12). The largest study was published by Makary *et al.* (170), reporting on a detection rate of nearly 25% and on an influence on survival by univariate analysis. Nakao *et al.* (171) found a comparable detection rate, but no influence on prognosis, whereas our own series on 80 patients demonstrated an influence on survival in a univariate analysis (160).

CONCLUSION AND PERSPECTIVES

The first reports on the cytological detection of disseminated tumor cells were published over 25 years ago. Nowadays, technical development allows the detection with an increased sensitivity. At present, immunocytochemical assays are regarded as the standard for the detection in bone marrow. The greater sensitivity of the molecular biological assays may have the potential to increase the detection rates, especially in the blood.

This overview over the detection of disseminated tumor cells in colorectal, gastric and pancreatic carcinoma demonstrates, that there are major differences between disseminated tumor cells in these three carcinomas and between the compartments in which they are detected. Detection rates and prognostic impact depend first on the kind of tumor and the compartment, but also on the methods and markers used, as well as the patient selection. Therefore, a definitive answer to the question of whether disseminated tumor cells in colorectal, gastric or pancreatic carcinoma are of prognostic relevance cannot be given at present.

In further studies, we will need to think of methodical standardization and, additionally, of comparable groups of patients. Larger groups of patients are required for multivariate analyses to prove the independence of the prognostic influence of the detection of disseminated tumor cells. The studies performed so far demonstrate, that the analyses of disseminated tumor cells in gastrointestinal carcinoma patients can help to improve the staging of these patients, and if further results can confirm the prognostic impact of one or more compartments, clinical consequences will be drawn.

Patients with proven disseminated tumor at the time of primary operation will have to receive adjuvant therapies, depending on the type of tumor and on further criteria, which have to be evaluated.

Additionally, the biology of early and occult tumor cell dissemination is so far not completely understood and requires further investigations. As recurrences are sometimes seen after a period of years, it is likely that disseminated cells can persist in a dormant state for prolonged periods. There is some evidence that these cells cannot be reached by conventional chemotherapy, but might be targeted by antibody-based adjuvant cancer therapies (175–178).

One problem that has to be overcome is the heterogeneity of solid tumors, since it limits the likelihood of removal of all disseminated cells. An individualized characterization of the tumor cells might be one solution (179), but this does not appear practicable in daily routine. It might be more efficient to use a cocktail of antibodies for such purposes.

All these aspects have to be evaluated further in studies considering methodical aspects (standard protocols (182), new marker genes, quantitative PCR, etc.), cell characterization, prognostic impact, and new adjuvant therapeutic approaches but will certainly lead to improvements in the treatment of gastrointestinal carcinoma in the future.

Acknowledgment

This work was supported by the "Hensel-Stiftung", a grant of the Medical Faculty of the University of Kiel (IZKF) and further by the "Krebsgesellschaft Schleswig-Holstein."

REFERENCES

1. Heald RJ, Moran BJ, Ryall RD, Sexton R, MacFarlane JK. Rectal cancer. The Basingstoke experience of total mesorectal excision, 1978–1997. Arch Surg. 1998; 133: 894–99.
2. Lehnert T, Herfarth C. Multimodale Therapie des Rectumcarcinoms. Chirurg. 1998; 69: 384–92.
3. Wittekind CH, Meyer HJ, Bootz F. TNM-Klassifikation maligner Tumoren. 6. Auflage 2002, Springer Verlag, Berlin, Heidelberg, New York.
4. Burchill SA, Lewis IJ, Selby P. Improved methods using the reverse transcriptase polymerase chain reaction to detect tumor cells. Br J Cancer. 1999; 79: 971–77.
5. Burchill SA, Selby PJ. Molecular detection of low-level disease in patients with cancer. J Pathol. 2000; 190: 6–14.
6. Juhl H, Kalthoff H, Krüger U, Schott A, Schreiber HW, Henne-Bruns D, Kremer B. Immunzytologischer Nachweis disseminierter Tumorzellen in der Bauchhöhle und im Knochenmark von Pankreaskarzinom-Patienten. Chirurg. 1994; 65: 1111–15.
7. Palmieri G, Strazzullo M, Ascierto PA, Satriano SM, Daponte A, Castello G. Polymerase chain reaction-based detection of circulating melanoma cells as an effective marker of tumor progression. Melanoma Cooperative Group. J Clin Oncol. 1999; 17: 304–11.
8. Pantel K, Riethmüller G. Methods for detection of micrometastatic carcinoma cells in bone marrow, blood and lymph nodes. Onkologie. 1995; 18: 394–401.
9. Pantel K, von Knebel Doeberitz M, Izbicki JR, Riethmüller G. Disseminierte Tumorzellen: Diagnostik, prognostische Relevanz, Phänotypisierung und therapeutische Strategien. Chirurg. 1997; 68: 1241–50.
10. Pantel K, Schlimok G, Angstwurm M, Weckermann D, Schmaus W, Gath H, Passlick B, Izbicki JR, Riethmüller G. Methodological analysis of immunocytochemical screening for disseminated epithelial tumor cells in bone marrow. J Hematother. 1994; 3: 165–73.
11. Braun S, Hepp F, Sommer HL, Pantel K. Tumor-antigen heterogeneity of disseminated breast cancer cells: implications for immunotherapy of minimal residual disease. Int J Cancer. 1999; 84:1–5.

12. Kell MR, Winter DC, O'Sullivan GC, Shanahan F, Redmond HP. Biological behaviour and clinical implications on micrometastases. Br J Surg. 2000; 87: 1629–39.
13. Klein CA, Schmidt-Kittler O, Sachardt JA, Pantel K, Speicher MR, Riethmüller G. Comparative genomic hybridization, loss of heterozygosity, and DNA sequence analysis of single cells. Proc Natl Acad Sci USA. 1999; 96: 4494–99.
14. Noack F, Schmitt M, Bauer J, Helmecke D, Kruger W, Thorban S, Sandherr M, Kuhn W, Graeff H, Harbeck N. A new approach to phenotyping disseminated tumor cells: methodological advances and clinical implications. Int J Biol Markers. 2000; 15: 100–4.
15. Jung R, Krüger W, Hosch S, Holweg M, Kröger N, Gutensohn K, Wagener C, Neumaier M, Zander AR. Specificity of reverse transcriptase polymerase chain reaction assays designed for the detection of circulating cancer cells is influenced by cytokines in vivo and in vitro. Br J Cancer. 1998; 78: 1194–98.
16. Raj GV, Moreno JG, Gomella LG. Utilization of polymerase chain reaction technology in the detection of solid tumors. Cancer. 1998; 82: 1419–42.
17. Johnson PW, Burchill SA, Selby PJ. The molecular detection of circulating tumor cells. Br J Cancer. 1995; 72: 268–76.
18. Lambrechts AC, van't Veer LJ, Rodenhuis S. The detection of minimal numbers of contaminating epithelial tumor cells in blood or bone marrow: use, limitations and future of RNA-based methods. Ann Oncol. 1998; 9: 1269–76.
19. Soeth E, Röder C, Juhl H, Krüger U, Kremer B, Kalthoff H. The detection of disseminated tumor cells in bone marrow from colorectal-cancer patients by a cytokeratin-20-specific nested reverse-transcriptase-polymerase-chain reaction is related to the stage of disease. Int J Cancer. 1996; 69: 278–82.
20. Krüger W, Jung R, Kröger N, Gutensohn K, Fiedler W, Neumaier M, Jänicke F, Wagener C, Zander AR. Sensitivity of assays designed for the detection of disseminated epithelial tumor cells is influenced by cell separation methods. Clin Chemistry. 2000; 46:435–36.
21. Neumaier M, Gerhard M, Wagener C. Diagnosis of micrometastases by the amplification of tissue-specific genes. Gene. 1995; 159: 43–47.
22. Denis MG, Lipart C, Leborgne J, LeHur PA, Galmiche JP, Denis M, Ruud E, Truchaud A, Lustenberger P. Detection of disseminated tumor cells in peripheral blood of colorectal cancer patients. Int J Cancer. 1997; 74: 540–44.
23. Martin VM, Siewert C, Scharl A, Harms T, Heinze R, Ohl S, Radbruch A, Miltenyl S, Schmitz J. Immunomagnetic enrichment of disseminated epithelial tumor cells from peripheral blood by MACS. Exp Hematol. 1998; 26: 252–64.
24. Naume B, Borgen E, Nesland JM, Beiske K, Gilen E, Renolen A, Ravnas G, Quist H, Karesen R, Kvalheim G. Increased sensitivity for detection of micrometastatases in bone marrow/ peripheral blood stem-cell products from breast-cancer patients by negative immunomagnetic separation. Int J Cancer. 1998; 78: 556–60.
25. Slade MJ, Smith BM, Sinnett HD, Cross NC, Coombes RC. Quantitative polymerase chain reaction for the detection of micrometastases in patients with breast cancer. J Clin Oncol. 1999; 17: 870–79.
26. Bustin SA, Gyselman VG, Williams NS, Dorudi S. Detection of cytokeratins 19/20 and Guanylyl Cyclase C in peripheral blood of colorecal cancer patients. Br J Cancer. 1999; 79: 1813–20.
27. Ghossein RA, Bhattacharya S, Rosain J. Molecular detection of micrometastases and circulating tumor cells in solid tumors. Clin Cancer Res. 1999; 5: 1950–60.
28. Goeminne JC, Guillaume T, Symann M. Pitfalls in the detection of disseminated non-hematological tumor cells. Ann Oncol. 2000; 11: 785–92.

29. Hayashi N, Ito I, Yanagisawa A, Kato Y, Nakamori S, Imaoka S, Watanabe H, Ogawa M, Nakamura K. Genetic diagnosis of lymph-node metastasis in colorectal cancer. Lancet. 1995; 345: 1257–59.
30. Heiss MM, Allgayer H, Gruetzner KU, Babic R, Jauch KW, Schildberg FW. Clinical value of extended biologic staging by bone marrow micrometastases and tumor-associated proteases in gastric cancer. Ann Surg. 1997; 226: 736–45.
31. Maguire D, O'Sullivan GC, Collins JK, Morgan J, Shanahan F. Bone marrow metastases and gastrointestinal cancer detection and significance. Am J Gastroenterol. 2000; 95: 1644–51.
32. Müller P, Schlimok G. Bone marrow 'micrometastases' of epithelial tumors: detection and clinical relevance. J Cancer Res Clin Oncol. 2000; 126: 607–18.
33. Pantel K, Cote RJ, Fodstad Ø. Detection and clinical importance of micrometastatic disease. J Natl Cancer I. 1999; 91: 1113–24.
34. Tsavallas G, Patel H, Allen-Mersh TG. Detection and clinical significance of occult tumor cells in colorectal cancer. Br J Surg. 2001; 88: 1307–20.
35. Von Knebel Doeberitz M, Koch M, Weitz J, Herfarth C. Diagnostik und Bedeutung der 'Minimal Residual Disease' bei Patienten mit kolorektalem Karzinom. Zentralbl Chir. 2000; 125 (Suppl 1): 15–19.
36. Sasaki M, Watanabe H, Jass JR, Ajioka Y, Kobayashi M, Matsuda K, Hatakeyama K. Occult lymph node metastases detected by cytokeratin immunohistochemistry predict recurrence in 'node-negative' colorectal cancer. J Gastroenterol. 1997; 32: 758–64.
37. Yonemura Y, Fujimura T, Ninomiya I, Kim BS, Bandou E, Sawa T, Kinoshita K, Endo Y, Sugiyama K, Sasaki T. Prediction of peritoneal micrometastasis by peritoneal lavaged cytology and reverse transcriptase-polymerase chain reaction for matrix metalloproteinase-7 mRNA. Clin Cancer Res. 2001; 7: 1647–53.
38. Adell G, Boeryd B, Franund B, Sjödahl R, Hakansson L. Occurrence and prognostic importance of micrometastases in regional lymph nodes in Duke's B coloretal carcinoma: an immunohistochemical study. Eur J Surg. 1996; 162: 637–42.
39. Cutait R, Alves VAF, Lopes LC, Cutait DE, Boges JLA, Singer J da Silva H, Goffi FS. Restaging of colorectal cancer based on the identification of lymph node micrometastases through immunoperoxidase staining of CEA and cytokeratins. Dis Colon Rectum. 1991; 34: 917–20.
40. Nakanishi Y, Ochiai A, Yamauchi Y, Moriya Y, Yoshumura K, Hirohashi S. Clinical implications of lymph node micrometastases in patients with colorectal cancers. A case control study. Oncology 1999; 57: 276–80.
41. Öberg A, Stenling R, Tavelin B, Lindmark G. Are lymph node micrometastases of any clinical significance in Dukes stages A and B colorectal cancer? Dis Colon Rectum. 1998; 41: 1244–49.
42. Greenson JK, Isenhart CE, Rice R, Mojzik C, Houchens D, Martin EW Jr. Identification of occult micrometastases in pericolic lymph nodes of Duke's B colorectal cancer patients using monoclonal antibodies against cytokeratin and CC49. Correlation with long-term survival. Cancer. 1994; 73: 563–69.
43. Liefers GJ, Cleton-Jansen AM, van de Velde H, Hermans J, van Krieken JHJM, Cornelisse CJ, Tollenaar RAEM. Micrometastases and survival in stage II colorectal cancer. N Engl J Med. 1998; 339: 223–28.
44. Makin CA, Bobrow LG, Nicholls RJ. Can immunohistology improve detection of lymph-node metastases in large-bowel cancer? Dis Colon Rectum. 1989; 32: 99–102.
45. Davidson BR, Sams VR, Styles J, Deane C, Boulos PB. Detection of occult nodal metastases in patients with colorectal carcinoma. Cancer. 1990; 65: 967–70.

46. Haboubi NY, Cark P, Kaftan SM, Schofield PF. The importance of combining xylene clearance and immunohistochemistry in the accurate staging of colorectal carcinoma. J R Soc Med. 1992; 85: 386–88.
47. Jeffers MD, O'Dowd GM, Mulcahy H, Staag M, O'Donoghue DP, Toner M. The prognostic significance of immunohistochemically detected lymph nodes micrometastases in colorectal carcinoma. J Pathol. 1994; 172: 183–87.
48. Nicholson AG, Marks CG, Cook MG. Effect on lymph node status of triple levelling and immunohistochemistry with CAM 5.2 on node negative colorectal carcinomas. Gut. 1994; 35: 1447–48.
49. Cote RJ, Houchens DP, Hitchcock CL, Saad AD, Nines RG, Greenson JK, Schneebaum S, Arnold MW, Martin EW. Intraoperative detection of occult colon cancer micrometastases using 125 I-radiolabeled monoclonal antibody CC49. Cancer. 1996; 77: 613–20.
50. Broll R, Schauer V, Schimmelpenning H, Strik M, Woltmann A, Best R, Bruch H-P, Duchrow M. Prognostic relevance of occult tumor cells in lymph nodes of colorectal carcinomas: an immunohistochemical study. Dis Colon Rectum. 1997; 40: 1465–71.
51. Hitchcock CL, Sampsel J, Young DC, Martin EW, Arnold MW. Limitations with light microscopy in the detection of colorectal cancer cells. Dis Colon Rectum. 1999; 42: 1046–52.
52. Yasuda K, Adachi Y, Shiraishi N, Yamaguchi K, Hirabayashi Y, Kitano S. Pattern of lymph node micrometastases and prognosis of patients with colorectal cancer. Ann Surg Oncol. 2001; 8: 300–4.
53. Mori M, Mimori K, Inoue H, Barnard GF, Tsuji K, Nanbara S, Ueo H, Akiyoshi T. Detection of cancer micrometastases in lymph nodes by reverse transcriptase-polymerase chain reaction. Cancer Res. 1995; 55: 3417–20.
54. Futamura M, Takagi Y, Koumura H, Kida H, Tanemura H, Shimokawa K, Saji S. Spread of colorectal cancer micrometastases in regional lymph nodes by reverse transcriptase-polymerase chain reactions for carcinoembryonic antigen and cytokeratin 20. J Surg Oncol. 1998; 68: 34–40.
55. Mori M, Mimori K, Ueo H, Tsuji K, Shiraishi T, Barnard GF, Sugimachi K, Akiyoshi T. Clinical significance of molecular detection of carcinoma cells in lymph nodes and peripheral blood by reverse transcriptation-polymerase chain reaction in patients with gastrointestinal or breast carcinomas. J Clin Oncol. 1998; 16: 128–32.
56. Rosenberg R, Hoos A, Mueller J, Nekarda H. Impact of cytokeratin-20 and carcinoembryonic antigen mRNA detection by RT-PCR in regional lymph nodes of patients with colorectal cancer. Br J Cancer. 2000; 83: 1323–29.
57. Miyake Y, Yamamoto H, Fujiwara Y, Ohue M, Sugita Y, Tomiita N, Sekimoto M, Matsuura N, Shiozaki H, Monden M. Extensive micrometastases to lymph nodes as a marker for rapid recurrence of colorectal cancer: a study of lymphatic mapping. Clin Cancer Res. 2001; 7:1350–57.
58. Gunn J, McCall JL, Yun K, Wright PA. Detection of micrometastases in colorectal cancer patients by K19 and K20 reverse-transcription polymerase chain reaction. Lab Invest. 1996; 75: 611–16.
59. Dorudi S, Kinrade E, Marshall NC, Freakins R, Williams NS, Bustin SA. Genetic detection of lymph node micrometastases in patients with colorectal cancer. Br J Surg. 1998; 85: 98–100.
60. Merrie AE, Yun K, van Rij AM, McCall JL. Detection and significance of minimal residual disease in colorectal cancer. Histol Histopathol. 1999; 14: 561–69.
61. Weitz J, Kienle P, Magener A, Koch M, Schröel A, Willeke F, Autschbach F, Lacroix J, Lehnert T, Herfarth C, von Knebel Doeberitz M. Detection of disseminated colorectal cancer cells in lymph nodes, blood and bone marrow. Clin Cancer Res. 1999; 5: 1830–36.

62. Yun K, Merrie AEH, Gunn J, Phillips LV, McCall JL. Keratin 20 is a specific marker of submicroscopic lymph node metastases in colorectal cancer: validation by K-RAS mutations. J Pathol. 2000; 191: 21–26.
63. Sanchez-Cespedes M, Esteller M, Hibi K, Cope FO, Westra W, Piantadosi S, Herman JG, Jen J, Sidransky D. Molecular detection of neoplastic cells in lymph nodes of metastatic colorectal cancer patients predicts recurrence. Clin Cancer Res. 1999; 5: 2450–54.
64. Clarke GA, Ryan E, Crowe JP, O'Keane JC, MacMathúna P. Tumor-derived mutated K-ras codon 12 expression in regional lymph nodes of stage II colorectal cancer patients is not associated with increased risk of cancer-related death. Int J Colorectal Dis. 2001; 16: 108–11.
65. Bernini A, Spencer M, Frizelle S, Maoff RD, Wilmtt LD, McComick SR, Niehans GA, Ho SB, Kratzke RA. Evidence for colorectal cancer micrometastases using reverse transcriptase-polymerase chain reaction analysis of MUC2 in lymph nodes. Cancer Detect Prev. 2000; 24: 72–79.
66. Wong LS, Cantrill JE, Odogwu S, Morris AG, Fraser IA. Detection of circulating tumor cells and nodal metastasis by reverse transcriptase-polymerase chain reaction technique. Br J Surg. 1997; 84: 834–39.
67. Ichikawa Y, Ishikawa T, Momiyama N, Yamaguchi S, Masui H, Hasegawa S, Chishima T, Takimto A, Kitamura H, Akitaya T, Hosokawa T, Mitsuhashi M, Shimada H. Detection of regional lymph node metastases in colon cancer by using RT-PCR for matrix metalloproteinase 7, matrilysin. Clin Exp Metastasis. 1998; 16: 3–8.
68. Waldman SA, Cagir B, Rakinic J, Fry RD, Goldstein SD, Isenberg G, Barber M, Biswas S, Minimo C, Palazzo J, Park PK, Weinberg D. Use of Guanylyl Cylase C for detecting micrometastases in lymph nodes of patients with colon cancer. Dis Colon Rectum. 1998; 41: 310–15.
69. Aihara T, Fujiwara Y, Miyake Y, Okami J, Okada Y, Iwao K, Sugita Y, Tomita N, Sakon M, Shiozaki H, Monden M. Mammaglobin B gene as a novel marker for lymph node micrometastases in patients with abdominal cancers. Cancer Lett. 2000; 150: 79–84.
70. Schlimok G, Funke I, Holzmann B, Göttlinger G, Schmidt G, Häuser H, Swierkot S, Warnecke HH, Schneider B, Koprowski H, Riethmüller G. Micrometastatic cells in bone marrow: in vitro detection with anticytokeratin and in vivo labeling with anti-17–1A monoclonal antibodies. Proc Natl Acad Sci USA. 1987; 84: 8672–76.
71. Lindemann F, Schlimok G, Dirschedl P, Witte J, Riethmüller G. Prognostic significance of micrometastatic tumor cells in bone marrow of colorectal cancer patients. Lancet. 1992; 340: 685–89.
72. Leinung S, Würl P, Weiss CL, Röder I, Schönfelder M. Cytokeratin-positive cells in bone marrow in comparison with other prognostic factors in colon carcinoma. Langenbeck's Arch Surg. 2000; 385: 337–43.
73. Jung R, Petersen K, Krüger W, Wolf M, Wagener C, Zander A, Neumaier M. Detection of micrometastasis by cytokeratin 20 RT-PCR is limited due to stable background transcription in granulocytes. Br J Cancer. 1999; 81: 870–73.
74. Pelkey TJ, Frierson HF Jr, Bruns DE. Molecular and immunological detection of circulating tumor cells and micrometastases from solid tumors. Clin Chem. 1996; 42: 1369–81.
75. Gerhard M, Juhl H, Kalthoff H, Schreiber HW, Wagener C, Neumaier M. Specific detection of carcinoembryonic antigen-expressing tumor cells in bone marrow aspirates by polymerase chain reaction. J Clin Oncol. 1994; 12: 725–29.
76. Vogel I, Soeth E, Röder C, Kremer B, Henne-Bruns D, Kalthoff H. Multivariate analysis reveals RT-PCR-detected tumour cells in the blood and/or bone marrow of patients with colorectal carcinoma as an independent prognostic factor. Eur J Clin Oncol. 2000; 26: 281.
77. Schneider BM, Schlimok G, Riethmüller G, Witte J. Knochenmarksmikrometastasen bei kolorektalen Karzinomen. Fortschr Med. 1989; 107: 59–63.

78. Schlimok G, Funke I, Bock B, Schweiberer B, Witte J, Riethmüller G. Epithelial tumor cells in bone marrow of patients with colorectal cancer: immunocytochemical detection, phenotypic characterization, and prognostic significance. J Clin Oncol. 1990: 8: 831–37.
79. O'Sullivan GC, Collins JK, O'Brien F, Crowley B, Murphy K, Lee G, Shanahan F. Micrometastases in bone marrow of patients undergoing 'curative' surgery for gastrointesti nal cancer. Gastroenterology. 1995; 109: 1535–40.
80. Broll R, Lembcke K, Stock C, Zingler M, Duchrow M, Schimmelpenning H, Strik M, Müller G, Kujath P, Bruch HP. Tumorzelldissemination in das Knochenmark und in die Peritonealhöhle. Langenbeck Arch Chir. 1996; 381: 51–58.
81. Cohen AM, Garin-Chesa P, Hanson M, Weyhrauch K, Kemeny N, Fong Y, Paty P, Welt S, Old L. In vitro detection of occult bone marrow metastases in patients with colorectal cancer hepatic metastases. Dis Colon Rectum. 1998; 41:1112–15.
82. Schott A, Vogel I, Krueger U, Kalthoff H, Schreiber HW, Schmiegel W, Henne-Bruns D, Kremer B, Juhl H. Isolated tumor cells are frequently detectable in the peritoneal cavity of gastric and colorectal cancer patients and serve as a new prognostic marker. Ann Surg. 1998; 227: 372–79.
83. Litle VR, Warren RS, Moore II D, Pallavicini MG. Molecular cytogenetic analysis of cytokeratin 20-labeled cells in primary tumors and bone marrow aspirates from colorectal carcinoma patients. Cancer. 1997; 79:1664–70.
84. Soeth E, Vogel I, Röder C, Juhl H, Marxsen J, Krüger U, Henne-Bruns D, Kremer B, Kalthoff H. Comparative analysis of bone marrow and venous blood isolates from gastrointestinal cancer patients for the detection of disseminated tumor cells using reverse transcription PCR. Cancer Res. 1997; 57: 3106–10.
85. Weitz J, Koch M, Kienle P, Schrodel A, Willeke F, Brenner A, Lehnert T, Herfarth C, von Knebel Doeberitz M. Detection of hematogenic tumor cell dissemination in patients undergoing resection of liver metastases of colorectal cancer. Ann Surg. 2000; 232: 66–72.
86. Hardingham JE, Kotasek D, Sage RE, Eaton MC, Pascoe VH, Dobrovic A. Detection of circulating tumor cells in colorectal cancer by immunobead-PCR is a sensitive prognostic marker for relapse of disease. Mol Med. 1995; 1: 789–94.
87. Hardingham JE, Hewett PJ, Sage RE, Finch JL, Nuttall JD, Kotasek D, Dobrovic A. Molecular detection of blood-borne epithelial cells in colorectal cancer patients and in patients with benign bowel disease. Int J Cancer. 2000; 89: 8–13.
88. Khan ZAJ, Jonas SK, Le-Marer N, Patel H, Wharton RQ, Tarragona A, Ivision A, Allen-Mersh TG. p53 mutations in primary and metastatic tumors and circulating tumor cells from colorectal carcinoma patients. Clin Cancer Res. 2000; 6: 3499–504.
89. Jonas S, Windeatt S, O-Boateng A, Fordy C, Allen-Mersh TG. Identification of carcinoembryonic antigen-producing cells circulating in the blood of patients with colorectal carcinoma by reverse transcriptase polymerase chain reaction. Gut. 1996; 39: 717–21.
90. Mori M, Mimori K, Ueo H, Karimine N, Barnard GF, Sugimachi K, Akiyoshi T. Molecular detection of circulating solid carcinoma cells in the peripheral blood: the concept of early systemic disease. Int J Cancer. 1996; 68: 739–43.
91. Castells A, Boix L, Bessa X, Gargallo L, Pique JM. Detection of colonic cells in peripheral blood of colorectal cancer patients by means of reverse transcriptase and polymerase chain reaction. Br J Cancer. 1998; 78: 1368–72.
92. Ko Y, Klinz M, Totzke G, Gouni-Berthold I, Sachinidis A, Vetter H. Limitations of the reverse transcription-polymerase chain reaction method for the detection of carcinoembryonic antigen-positive tumor cells in peripheral blood. Clin Cancer Res. 1998; 4: 2141–46.
93. Noh YH, Im G, Ku JH, Lee YS, Ahn MJ. Detection of tumor cell contamination in peripheral blood by RT-PCR in gastrointestinal cancer patients. J Korean Med Sci. 1999; 14: 623–28.

94. Taniguchi T, Makino M, Suzuki K, Kaibara N. Prognostic significance of reverse transcriptase-polymerase chain reaction measurement of carcinoembryonic antigen mRNA levels in tumor drainage blood and peripheral blood of patients with colorectal carcinoma. Cancer. 2000; 89: 970–76.
95. Piva MG, Navaglia F, Basso D, Fogar P, Roveroni G, Gallo N, Zambon C-F, Pedrazzoli S, Plebani M. CEA mRNA identification in peripheral blood is feasible for colorectal, but not for gastric or pancreatic cancer staging. Oncology. 2000; 59: 323–28.
96. Guadagni F, Kantor J, Aloe S, Carone MD, Spila A, D'Alessandro R, Abbolito MR, Cosimelli M, Graziano F, Carboni F, Carlini S, Perri P, Sciarretta F, Greiner JW, Kashmiri SVS, Steinberg SM, Roselli M, Schlom J. Detection of blood-borne cells in colorectal cancer patients by nested reverse transcription-polymerase chain reaction for carcinoembryonic antigen messenger RNA: longitudinal analyses and demonstration of its potential importance as an adjunct to multiple serum markers. Cancer Res. 2001; 61: 2523–32.
97. Bessa X, Elizalde JI, Boix L, Pinol V, Lacy AM, Salo J, Pique JM, Castells A. Lack of prognostic influence of circulating tumor cells in peripheral blood of patients with colorectal cancer. Gastroenterology. 2001; 120: 1084–92.
98. Masson D, Denis MG, Lustenberger P. Limitations of CD44v6 amplification for the detection of tumour cells in the blood of colorectal cancer patients. Br J Cancer. 2000; 82: 1283–89.
99. Burchill SA, Bradbury MF, Pittman K, Southgate J, Smith B, Selby P. Detection of epithelial cancer cells in peripheral blood by reverse transcriptase-polymerase chain reaction. Br J Cancer. 1995; 71: 278–81.
100. Nakamori S, Kameyama M, Furukawa H, Takeda O, Sugai S, Imaoka S, Nakamura Y. Genetic detection of colorectal cancer cells in circulation and lymph nodes. Dis Colon Rectum. 1997; 40 (Suppl.): S29–S36.
101. Funaki NO, Tanaka J, Itami A, Kasamatsu T, Ohshio G, Onodera H, Monden K, Okino T, Imamura M. Detection of colorectal carcinoma cells in circulating peripheral blood by reverse transcription-polymerase chain reaction targeting cytokeratin-20 mRNA. Life Sci 1997; 60: 643–52.
102. Funaki NO, Tanaka J, Ohshio G, Onodera H, Maetani S, Imamura M. Cytokeratin 20 mRNA in peripheral venous blood of colorectal carcinoma patients. Br J Cancer. 1998; 77: 1327–32.
103. Wyld DK, Selby P, Perren TJ, Jonas SK, Allen-Mersh TG, Wheeldon J, Burchill SA. Detection of colorectal cancer cells in peripheral blood by reverse-transcriptase polymerase chain reaction for cytokeratin 20. Int J Cancer. 1998; 79: 288–93.
104. Weitz J, Kienle P, Lacroix J, Willeke F, Brenner A, Lehnert T, Herfarth C, von Knebel Doeberitz M. Dissemination of tumor cells in patients undergoing surgery for colorectal cancer. Clin Cancer Res. 1998; 4: 343–48.
105. Champelovier P, Mongelard F, Seigneurin D. CK 20 gene expression: technical limits for the detection of circulating tumor cells. Anticancer Res. 1999; 19: 2073–78.
106. Chausovsky G, Luchansky M, Fier A, Shapira J, Gottfried M, Novis B, Bogelman G, Zemer R, Zimlichman S, Klein A. Expression of cytokeratin 20 in the blood of patients with disseminated carcinoma of the pancreas, colon, stomach and lung. Cancer. 1999; 6: 2398–405.
107. Wharton RQ, Jonas SK, Glover C, Khan ZA, Klokouzas A, Quinn H, Henry M, Allen-Mersh TG. Increased detection of circulating tumor cells in the blood of colorectal carcinoma patients using two reverse transcription assays and multiple blood samples. Clin Cancer Res. 1999; 5: 4158–63.
108. Funaki NO, Tanaka J, Sugiyama T, Ohshio G, Nonaka A, Yotsumoto F, Furutani M, Imamura M. Perioperative quantitative analysis of cytokeratin 20 mRNA in peripheral venous blood of patients with colorectal adenocarcinoma. Oncol Rep. 2000; 7: 21–76.

109. Patel H, Le-Marer N, Wharton RQ, Khan ZAJ, Araia R, Henry MM, Allen-Mersh TG. Clearance of circulating tumour cells is greatest in tumours with the best prognosis. Br J Surg. 2000; 87: 630.
110. Yamaguchi K, Takagi Y, Aoki S, Futamura M, Saji S. Significant detection of circulating cancer cells in the blood by reverse transcriptase-polymerase chain reaction during colorectal cancer resection. Ann Surg. 2000; 232: 58–65.
111. Mathur P, Wharton RQ, Jonas SK, Saini S, Allen-Mersh TG. Relationship between tumor vascularity and circulating cancer cells in patients with colorectal carcinoma. EJSO. 2001; 27: 354–58.
112. Ambrose NS, MacDonald F, Young J, Thompson H, Keighley MR. Monoclonal antibody and cytological detection of free malignant cells in the peritoneal cavity during resection of colorectal cancer – can monoclonal antibodies do better? Eur J Surg Oncol. 1985; 15: 99–102.
113. Juhl H, Stritzel M, Wroblewski A, Henne-Bruns D, Kremer B, Schmiegel W, Neumaier M, Wagener C, Schreiber HW, Kalthoff H. Immunocytological detection of micrometastatic cells: comparative evaluation of findings in the peritoneal cavity and the bone marrow of gastric, colorectal and pancreatic cancer patients. Int J Cancer. 1994; 57: 330–35.
114. Broll R, Weschta M, Windhoevel U, Berndt S, Schwandner O, Roblick U, Schiedeck THK, Schimmelpenning H, Bruch HP, Duchrow M. Prognostic significance of free gastrointestinal tumor cells in peritoneal lavage detected by immunocytochemistry and polymerase chain reaction. Langenbeck's Arch Surg. 2001; 386: 285–92.
115. Harrison LE, Choe JK, Goldstein M, Meridian A, Kim SH, Clarke K. Prognostic significance of immunohistochemical micrometastases in node negative gastric cancer patients. J Surg Oncol. 2000; 73: 153–57.
116. Ikeguchi M, Cai J, Oka S, Gomyou Y, Tsujitani S, Maeta M, Kaibara N. Nuclear profiles of cancer cells reveal the metastatic potential of gastric cancer. J Pathol 2000; 192: 19–25.
117. Maehara Y, Yamamoto M, Oda S, Baba H, Kusumoto T, Ohno S, Ichiyoshi Y, Sugimachi K. Cytokeratin-positive cells in bone marrow for identifying distant micrometastasis of gastric cancer. Br J Cancer. 1996; 73: 83–87.
118. Fukagawa T, Sasako M, Mann GB, Sano T, Katai H, Maruyama K, Nakanishi Y, Shimoda T. Immunohistochemically detected micrometastases of the lymph nodes in patients with gastric carcinoma. Cancer. 2001; 92: 753–60.
119. Morgagni P, Saragoni L, Folli S, Gaudio M, Scarpi E, Bazzocchi F, Marras GA, Vio A. Lymph node micrometastases in patients with early gastric cancer: experiences with 139 patients. Ann Surg Oncol. 2001; 8: 170–74.
120. Saragoni L, Gaudio M, Morgagni P, Folli S, Bazzocchi F, Scarpi E, Saragoni A. Identification of occult micrometastases in patients with early gastric cancer using anti-cytokeratin monoclonal antibodies. Oncol Rep. 2000; 7: 535–39.
121. Stachura J, Zembala M, Heitzman J, Korabiowska M, Schauer A. Lymph node micrometastases in early gastric carcinoma alone inadequately reflect the new model of metastatic development. Pol J Pathol. 1998; 49: 155–57.
122. Kestlmeier R, Busch R, Fellbaum C, Boettcher K, Reich U, Siewert JR, Hoffler H. Incidence and prognostic significance of epitheloid cell reactions and microcarcinoses in regional lymph nodes in stomach carcinoma. Pathologe. 1997; 18: 124–30.
123. Siewert JR, Kestelmeier R, Busch R, Böttcher K, Roder JD, Müller J, Fellbaum C, Höfler H. Benefits of D2 lymph node dissection for patients with gastric cancer and pN0 and pN1 lymph node metastases. Br J Surg. 1996; 83: 1144–47.
124. Ishida K, Katsuyama T, Sugiyama A, Kawasaki S. Immunohistochemical evaluation of lymph node micrometastases from gastric carcinomas. Cancer. 1997; 79: 1069–76.

125. Nakajo A, Natsugoe S, Ishigami S, Matsumoto M, Nakashima S, Hokita S, Baba M, Takao S, Aikou T. Detection and prediction of micrometastasis in the lymph nodes of patients with pN0 gastric cancer. Ann Surg Oncol. 2001; 8: 158–62.
126. Cai J, Ikeguchi M, Maeta M, Kaibara N. Micrometastasis in lymph nodes and microinvasion of the muscularis propria in primary lesions of submucosal gastric cancer. Surgery. 2000; 127: 32–39.
127. Noguchi S, Hiratsuka M, Furukawa H, Aihara T, Kasugai T, Tamura S, Imaoka S, Koyama H, Iwanaga T. Detection of gastric cancer micrometastases in lymph nodes by amplification of keratin 19 mRNA with reverse transcriptase-polymerase chain reaction. Jpn J Cancer Res. 1996; 87: 650–54.
128. Aihara T, Noguchi S, Ishikawa O, Furukawa H, Hiratsuka M, Ohigashi H, Nakamori S, Monden M, Imaoka S. Detection of pancreatic and gastric cancer cells in peripheral and portal blood by amplification of keratin 19 mRNA with reverse transcriptase-polymerase chain reaction. Int J Cancer. 1997; 72: 408–11.
129. Okada Y, Fujiwara Y, Yamamoto H, Sugita Y, Yasuda T, Doki Y, Tamura S, Yano M, Shiozaki H, Matsuura N, Monden M. Genetic detection of lymph node micrometastases in patients with gastric carcinoma by multiple-marker reverse transcriptase-polymerase chain reaction assay. Cancer. 2001; 92: 2056–64.
130. Jauch KW, Heiss MM, Gruetzner U, Funke I, Pantel K, Babic R, Eissner HJ, Riethmüller G, Schildberg FW. Prognostic significance of bone marrow micrometastases in patients with gastric cancer. J Clin Oncol. 1996; 14: 1810–17.
131. Heiss MM, Allgayer H, Gruetzner KU, Funke I, Babic R, Jauch KW, Schildberg FW. Individual development and uPA-receptor expression of disseminated tumor cells in bone marrow: a reference to early systemic disease in solid cancer. Nat Med. 1995; 1: 1035–39.
132. Moll R, Löwe A, Laufer J, Franke WW. Cytokeratin 20 in human carcinomas. A new histodiagnostic marker detected by monoclonal antibodies. Am J Pathol. 1992; 140: 427–47.
133. Moll R, Zimbelmann R, Goldschmidt MD, Keith M, Laufer J, Kasper M, Koch PJ, Franke WW. The human gene encoding cytokeratin 20 and its expression during fetal development and in gastrointestinal carcinomas. Differentiation. 1993; 53: 75–93.
134. Schlimok G, Funke I, Pantel K, Strobel F, Lindemann F, Witte J, Riethmüller G. Micrometastatic tumor cells in bone marrow of patients with gastric cancer: methodological aspects of detection and prognostic significance. Eur J Cancer. 1991; 27: 1461–65.
135. O'Sullivan GC, Collins JK, Kelly J, Morgan J, Madden M, Shanahan F. Micrometastases: marker of metastatic potential or evidence of residual disease? Gut. 1997; 40: 512–15.
136. Funke I, Fries S, Rolle M, Heiss MM, Untch M, Bohmert H, Schildberg W, Jauch KW. Comparative analyses of bone marrow micrometastases in breast and gastric cancer. Int J Cancer. 1996; 65: 755–61.
137. Allgayer H, Heiss MM, Riesenberg R, Grutzner KU, Tarabichi A, Babic R, Schildberg FW. Urokinase plasminogen activator receptor (uPA-R): one potential characteristic of metastatic phenotypes in minimal residual disease. Cancer Res. 1997; 57: 1394–99.
138. Kerner T, Hauzenberger T, Jauch KW. Nachweis und Bedeutung der Tumorzelldissemination beim Magenkarzinom. Onkologe. 1998; 4: 294–300.
139. Liu F, Li J, Zhang J. Detection of micrometastases in the bone marrow in patients with gastric cancer. Zhonghua Wai Ke Za Zhi. 1995; 33: 554–56.
140. Funaki NO, Tanaka J, Itami A, Kasamatsu T, Ohshio G, Onodera H, Monden K, Okino T, Imamura M. Detection of colorectal carcinoma cells in circulating peripheral blood by reverse transcription-polymerase chain reaction targeting cytokeratin-20 mRNA. Life Sci. 1997; 60: 643–52.

141. Nishida S, Kitamura K, Ichikawa D, Koike H, Tani N, Yamagishi H. Molecular detection of disseminated cancer cells in the peripheral blood of patients with gastric cancer. Anticancer Res. 2000; 20: 2155–59.
142. Miyazono F, Takao S, Natsugoe S, Uchikura K, Kijima F, Aridome K, Shinchi H, Takashi A. Molecular detection of circulating cancer cells during surgery in patients with biliary-pancreatic cancer. Am J Surg. 1999; 117: 475–79.
143. Murphy PD, Wadhera V, Griffin SM, Burgess P, Farell D, Taylor I, Hair T, Clague MB, Griffith CD. Free peritoneal tumor cell identification in patients with gastric and colorectal cancer. J R Coll Surg Edinb. 1993; 38: 28–32.
144. Benevelo M, Mottolese M, Cosimelli M, Tedesco M, Giannarelli D, Vasselli S, Carlini M, Garofalo A, Natali PG. Diagnostic and prognostic value of peritoneal immunocytology in gastric cancer. J Clin Oncol. 1998; 16: 3406–11.
145. Imada T, Rino Y, Cyo H, Oshima T, Hatori S, Wakebe S, Kabara K, Shiozawa M, Takahashi M, Takanashi Y. The detection of microscopically disseminated cancer cells in the abdominal cavity by intraoperative lavage cytology combined with an immunocytochemical method in gastric cancer. Anticancer Res. 1999; 1: 4965–68.
146. Nekarda H, Gess C, Stark M, Mueller JD, Fink U, Schenk U, Siewert JR. Immunocytochemically detected free peritoneal tumour cells (FPTC) are a strong prognostic factor in gastric carcinoma. Br J Cancer. 1999; 79: 611–19.
147. Abe N, Wantanabe T, Toda H, Machida H, Suzuki K, Masaki T, Mori T, Sugiyama M, Atomi Y, Nakaya Y. Prognostic influence of carcinoembryonic antigen levels in peritoneal washes in patients with gastric cancer. Am J Surg. 2001; 181: 356–61.
148. Kodera Y, Yamamura Y, Shimizu Y, Torii A, Hirai T, Yasui K, Morimoto T, Kato T, Kito T, Tatematsu M. Prognostic value and clinical implications of disseminated cancer cells in the peritoneal cavity detected by reverse transcriptase-polymerase chain reaction and cytology. Int J Cancer. 1998; 79: 429–33.
149. Nakanishi H, Kodera Y, Yamamura Y, Tatematsu M. Rapid quantitative detection of free cancer cells in the peritoneal cavity of gastric cancer patients with real-time RT-PCR, and its prognostic significance. Gan To Kagaku Ryoho 2001; 28: 784–88.
150. Fujimura T, Ohta T, Kitagawa H, Fushida S, Nishimura GI, Yonemura Y, Elnemr A, Miwa K, Nakanuma Y. Trypsinogen expression and early detection for peritoneal dissemination in gastric cancer. J Surg Oncol. 1998; 69: 71–75.
151. Schuhmacher C, Becker KF, Reich U, Schenk U, Mueller J, Siewert JR, Hofler H. Rapid detection of mutated E-cadherin in peritoneal lavage specimens from patients with diffuse-type gastric carcinoma. Diagn Mol Pathol. 1999; 8: 66–70.
152. Mori N, Oka M, Hazama S, Iizuka N, Yamamoto K, Yoshino S, Tangoku A, Noma T, Hirose K. Detection of telomerase activity in peritoneal fluid from patients with gastric cancer using immunomagnetic beads. Br J Cancer. 2000; 83: 1026–32.
153. Hosch SB, Knoefel WT, Metz S, Stoecklein N, Niendorf A, Broelsch CE, Izbicki JR. Early lymphatic tumor cell dissemination in pancreatic cancer: frequency and prognostic significance. Pancreas. 1997; 15: 154–59.
154. Tamagawa E, Ueda M, Takahashi S, Sugano K, Uematsu S, Mukai M, Ogata Y, Kitajima M. Pancreatic lymph nodal and plexus micrometastases detected by enriched polymerase chain reaction and nonradioisotopic single-strand conformation polymorphism analysis: a new predictive factor for recurrent pancreatic carcinoma. Clin Cancer Res. 1997; 3: 2143–49.
155. Ridwelski K, Meyer F, Fahlke J, Kasper U, Roessner A, Lippert H. Stellenwert von Cytokeratin- und Ca19–9-Antigen im immunhistochemischen Nachweis disseminierter Tumorzellen in Lymphknoten beim Pankreaskarzinom. Chirurg. 2001; 72: 920–26.

156. Ando N, Nakao A, Nomoto S, Takeda S, Kaneko T, Kurokawa T, Nonami T, Takagi H. Detection of mutant k-ras in dissected paraaortic lymph nodes of patients with pancreatic adenocarcinoma. Pancreas. 1997; 15: 374–78.
157. Demeure MJ, Doffek KM, Komorowski RA, Wilson SD. Adenocarcinoma of the pancreas. Detection of occult metastases in regional lymph nodes by polymerase chain reaction-based assay. Cancer. 1998; 83: 1328–34.
158. Demeure MJ, Doffek KM, Komorowski RA, Redlich PN, Zhu Y, Eickson BA, Ritch PS, Pitt HA, Wilson SD. Molecular metastases in stage I pancreatic cancer: improved survival with adjuvant chemoradiation. Surgery. 1998; 124: 663–69.
159. Brown HM, Ahrendt SA, Komorrowski RA, Doffek KM, Wilson SD, Demeure MJ. Immunohistochemistry and molecular detection of nodal micrometastases in pancreatic cancer. J Surg Res. 2001; 95: 141–46.
160. Vogel I, Krüger U, Marxsen J, Soeth E, Kalthoff H, Henne-Bruns D, Kremer B, Juhl H. Disseminated tumor cells in pancreatic cancer patients detected by immunocytology: a new prognostic factor. Clin Cancer Res. 1999; 5: 593–99.
161. Thorban S, Roder JD, Pantel K, Siewert JR. Epithelial tumor cells in bone marrow of patients with pancreatic carcinoma detected by immunocytochemical staining. Eur J Cancer 1996; 32A: 363–65.
162. Thorban S, Roder JD, Siewert JR. Detection of micrometastasis in bone marrow of pancreatic cancer patients. Ann Oncol. 1999 10 (Suppl. 4): 111–13.
163. Roder JD, Thorban S, Pantel K, Siewert JR. Micrometastases in bone marrow: prognostic indicators for pancreatic cancer. World J Surg. 1999; 23: 888–91.
164. Z'graggen K, Centeno BA, Fernandez-del Castillo C, Jimenez RE, Werner J, Warshaw AL. Biological implications of tumor cells in blood and bone marrow of pancreatic cancer patients. Surgery. 2001; 129: 537–46.
165. Tada M, Omata M, Kawai S, Saishio H, Ohto M, Saikiri RK, Sninsky JJ. Detection of ras gene mutations in pancreatic juice and peripheral blood of patients with pancreatic adenocarcinoma. Cancer Res. 1993; 53: 2472–74.
166. Nomoto S, Nakao A, Kasai Y, Harada A, Nonami T, Takagi H. Detection of ras gene mutations in perioperative peripheral blood with pancreatic adenocarcinoma. Jpn J Cancer Res. 1996; 87: 793–97.
167. Miyazono F, Natsugoe S, Takao S, Tokuda K, Kijima F, Aridome K, Hokita S, Baba M, Eizuru Y, Aikou T. Surgical maneuvers enhance molecular detection of circulating tumor cells during gastric cancer surgery. Ann Surg. 2001; 233: 189–94.
168. Kuroki T, Tomiokas T, Tajima Y, Inoue K, Ikemastsu Y, Ichinose K, Furui J, Kanematsu T. Detection of the pancreas-specific gene in the peripheral blood of patients with pancreatic carcinoma. Br J Cancer. 1999; 81: 350–53.
169. Bilchik A, Miyashiro M, Kelly M, Kuo C, Fujiwara Y, Nakamori S, Monden M, Hoon DS. Molecular detection of metastatic pancreatic carcinoma cells using a multimarker reverse transcriptase-polymerase chain reaction assay. Cancer. 2000; 88:103–4.
170. Makary MA, Warshaw AL, Centeno BA, Willett CG, Rattner DW, Fernandez-del Castillo C. Implications of peritoneal cytology for pancreatic cancer management. Arch Surg. 1998; 133: 361–65.
171. Nakao A, Oshima K, Takeda S, Kaneko T, Kanazumi N, Inoue S, Nomoto S, Kawase Y, Kasuya H. Peritoneal washings cytology combined with immunocytochemical staining in pancreatic cancer. Hepatogastroenterology. 1999; 46: 2974–77.
172. Nomoto S, Nakao A, Kasai Y, Inoue S, Harada A, Nonami T, Takagi H. Peritoneal washing cytology combined with immunocytochemical staining and detecting mutant K-ras in pancreatic cancer: comparison of the sensitivity and availability of various methods. Pancreas. 1997; 14: 126–32.

173. Rall CJ, Rivera JA, Centeno BA, Fernandez-del Castillo C, Rattner DW, Warshaw AL, Rustgi AK. Peritoneal exfoliative cytology and Ki-ras mutation analysis in patients with pancreatic adenocarcinoma. Cancer Lett. 1995; 97: 203–11.
174. Inoue S, Nakao A, Kasai Y, Harada A, Nonami T, Takagi H. Detection of hepatic micrometastasis in pancreatic adenocarcinoma patients by two-stage polymerase chain reaction/restriction fragment length polymorphism analysis. Jpn J Cancer Res. 1995; 86: 626–30.
175. Maxwell-Amstrong CA, Durrant LG, Scholefield JH. Immunotherapy for colorectal cancer. Am J Surg. 1999; 177: 344–48.
176. Riethmüller G, Holz E, Schlimok G, Schmiegel W, Raab R, Hoffken K, Gruber R, Funke I, Pichlmaier H, Hirche H, Buggisch P, Witte J, Pichlmayr R. Monoclonal antibody therapy for resected Dukes' C colorectal cancer: 7-year outcome of a multicenter randomized trial. J Clin Oncol. 1998; 16: 1788–94.
177. Schlimok G, Pantel K, Loibner H, Fackler-Schwalbe I, Riethmüller G. Reduction of metastatic carcinoma cells in bone marrow by intravenously administered monoclonal antibody: towards a novel surrogate test to monitor adjuvant therapies of solid tumors. Eur J Cancer. 1995; 31A: 1799–1803.
178. Vermorken JB, Claessen AM, van Tinteren H, Gall HE, Ezinga R, Meijer S, Scheper RJ, Meijer CJ, Bloemena E, Ransom JH, Hanna MG, Jr, Pinedo HM. Active specific immunotherapy for stage II and stage III human colon cancer: a randomised trial. Lancet. 1999; 353: 345–50.
179. Putz E, Witter K, Offner S, Stosiek P, Zippelius A, Johnson J, Zahn R, Riethmüller G, Pantel K. Phenotypic characteristics of cell lines derived from disseminated cancer cells in bone marrow of patients with solid epithelial tumors: establishment of working models for human micrometastases. Cancer Res. 1999; 59: 241–48.
180. Funaki NO, Tanaka J, Kasamatsu T, Ohshio G, Hosotani R, Okino T, Imamura M. Identification of carcinoembryonic antigen mRNA in circulating peripheral blood of pancreatic carcinoma and gastric carcinoma patients. Life Sci 1996; 59: 2187–99.
181. Ikeguchi M, Fukuda K, Oka S, Hisamitsu K, Katano K, Tsujitani S, Kaibara N. Micro-lymph node metastasis and its correlation with cathepsin D expression in early gastric cancer. J Surg Oncol 2001; 77: 188–94.
182. Vlems FA, Ladanyi A, Gertler R, Rosenberg R, Diepstra JH, Röder C, Nekarda H, Molnar B, Tulassay Z, van Muijen GN, Vogel I. Reliability of quantitative reverse-transcriptase-PCR-based detection of tumour cells in the blood between different laboratories using a standardised protocol. Eur J Cancer 2003; 39: 388–96.

Chapter 9

MINIMAL RESIDUAL DISEASE IN MELANOMA

Petra Goldin-Lang, Ulrich Keilholz

Department of Medicine III, University Hospital Benjamin Franklin, Free University Berlin, Hindenburgdamm 30, 12200 Berlin, Germany

Abstract
A number of specific genes encoding for melanosomal proteins are selectively expressed in melanocytes and melanomas. For detection of circulating melanoma cells, the expression of the *tyrosinase* gene is most widely used. Several cohorts of melanoma patients from single institutions have been analyzed by various research groups for the presence of circulating melanoma cells in all stages of disease. The percentage of patients with evidence for occult tumor dissemination has been correlated with the stage of disease in several, but not all, reports. Two prospective analyses suggest that the PCR result is of prognostic value in melanoma. Several laboratories have found PCR evidence for circulating melanoma cells in the great majority of untreated patients with Stage IV disease, other groups have reported much lower frequencies. Taken together, there is a wide range of results. Methodological differences are likely to account for this discrepancy. With the availability of true quantitative real-time reverse transcriptase (RT)-PCR systems, accurate quantification of *tyrosinase* transcripts over a range of 1 to 10,000 tumor cells per milliliter of blood is possible. Quantitative real-time RT-PCR systems also dramatically improve quality control, since exact quantitation of housekeeping gene mRNA facilitates determination of sample quality. Two large clinical trials are currently under way within the EORTC and in the US to adequately determine the clinical usefulness of PCR detection of minimal residual disease in melanoma.

1. INTRODUCTION

Malignant melanoma accounts for 1% to 3% of all malignant tumors (1). Once disseminated beyond the regional lymph nodes, malignant melanoma is largely incurable, with a median survival of 4–6 months (2). Early identification of melanoma patients at risk for hematogenous spread of the disease would be desirable. Therefore, polymerase chain reaction (PCR) tests to detect circulating melanoma cells have been developed.

In principle, single tumor cells in the bone marrow, for instance, can be detected by immunohistological techniques. However, this method is not sufficiently sensitive to reliably monitor early metastasis or minimal residual disease,

K. Pantel (ed.), Micrometastasis, 173–183.

since only a very limited number of cells can be assayed at one time. For the detection of occult metastasis from melanoma cells, several marker genes have been used, including *tyrosinase*, a key enzyme in the melanin biosynthetic pathway, melanA/MART-1, a melanosomal protein of unknown function or the melanoma-associated antigen A (MAGE-A) genes.

One limitation of those reverse transcriptase (RT)-PCR assays was the inability to quantitate the transcript amount accurately. The recently developed TaqMan and Light Cycler techniques combine amplification, detection and quantification, and are (a) easy to handle, (b) very rapid, (c) reproducible and (d) suited for high throughput screening applications. The novel possibility of real-time PCR is changing this whole field of investigation in two ways. First, real-time PCR provides quantitative data on minimal residual disease, which may be more informative. Secondly, real-time PCR allows much more detailed analysis of sample quality.

2. PRINCIPAL PCR DETECTION METHODS

This chapter describes the principles of occult tumor cell detection using PCR, and summarizes the currently available clinical data from trials utilizing PCR-based techniques. RNA-based methods require active transcription of the gene of interest. Fortunately, a high transcript number from the gene of interest is usually present in a tumor cell. RNA-based detection, therefore, has the advantage of high sensitivity and of detecting primarily viable cells, although detection of unviable cells in the early stages of apoptosis is theoretically possible. The number of RNA copies of a gene in any particular tumor cell may, however, vary during the cell's life cycle or as a result of de-differentiation.

2.1 Qualitative PCR Assay

RT-PCR is a highly sensitive method for detecting rare tumor-cell derived mRNA, allowing the diagnosis of tumor dissemination at early stages. This information may have important prognostic and therapeutic implications because residual tumor cells that are below the limit of detection using standard diagnostic techniques are nevertheless associated with increased risk for overt clinical relapse (3).

First, the RNA is extracted from the sample and the mRNA is reverse-transcribed into cDNA. The gene of interest is then amplified using primers specific for that gene. Ideally, these primers should not amplify genomic DNA, which often contaminates the cDNA preparation. Amplification of a cDNA sequence without amplification of the genomic counterpart of this sequence can be achieved if one primer is interrupted by an intron in the genomic DNA. The intron will have been deleted during RNA processing and, therefore, will not interrupt the primer sequence in the cDNA version of the gene. Alternatively, primers can be chosen that flank an intron in the genomic sequence, thereby facilitating easy differentiation between a PCR product derived from genomic DNA and one derived from cDNA based on the size of the amplicon. If intron/exon boundaries are unknown or targeted genes are intron-less, it is necessary to treat the RNA with RNase-free DNase.

One limitation of RT-PCR assays was the inability to quantitate the transcript amount, information that would be of interest for monitoring tumor progression or assessing the response to therapy in patients who prior to treatment had PCR evidence for circulating tumor cells.

2.2 Semiquantitative PCR Assay

Previous investigations have attempted to quantify *tyrosinase* transcripts using either serially diluted and differently sized competitor target molecules (4, 5, 6) or Southern blot analyses with a standardization to the expression of a housekeeping gene (7). Competitive PCR with a heterologous DNA (PCR MIMIC) as an internal standard was used. The method was validated by demonstration of similar amplification efficiencies for both molecules and by accurate quantitation of an artificial fourfold difference in the level of *tyrosinase* mRNA. The ratio of amplified target to amplified standard (at/as ratio) was determined (6). Alternatively, our groups developed a semiquantitative assessment to detect and quantitate circulating tumor cells by comparing the amount of RNA equivalent to *tyrosinase* mRNA content in a defined number of SK-mel 28 cell line (7, 8, 9). This latter principle is similar to the real-time PCR assays described below.

Both of these semiquantitative assays reside on close-to-end-point quantitation of transcript amounts, which is prone to influence PCR by rate-limiting reagents and product inhibition.

2.3 Real-time PCR

Real time RT-PCR offers for the first time the possibility to quantify templates rapidly and rather accurately using crossing points which mark the early exponential phase. This technique makes quantification much more precise and reproducible, because at the beginning of the exponential phase none of the reagents is rate limiting and only minimal inhibitory effects occur.

Using real-time PCRs, post-PCR steps are no longer necessary. PCR products are detected either by a dual labeled TaqMan probe with a reporter (FAM) and a quencher dye (TAMRA) at the 5′ and 3′- end or two Light Cycler hybridization probes labeled with a donor (Fluorescin) or acceptor fluorophore (LC Red 605/705) at the 3′ or 5′- end annealing to the target sequence in close proximity. Fluorescence signals arise by fluorescence energy transfer between donor and acceptor fluorophore (FRET) during primer annealing (Light Cycler probes) or by separating the reporter dye due to the 5′-nuclease activity of the Taq polymerase during elongation (TaqMan probe). Fluorescence signals are proportional to the initial number of target cDNA and are plotted versus crossing points which mark the cycle number when fluorescence becomes significantly different from baseline signal.

The transcript amount is calculated from the linear regression of a standard curve received by serial dilutions of (a) marker-specific PCR products, (b) marker expressing cell lines, (c) plasmids harboring the desired marker sequence or (d) recombinant plasmid derived *in vitro* transcripts. The relative amount of marker transcript-derived amplicons is expressed as ratio: marker – by housekeeping-gene transcripts. Normalization is important to compensate for differences in RNA and cDNA quality (sample to sample variation). Housekeeping genes are usually used for normalization because they are expected to be expressed at a constant level among different tissues and at all stages of development uneffected by experimental treatment. With the Light Cycler technique, PCR products can also be detected by Sybr Green which binds to nascent double-stranded DNA. This results in an increase in fluorescence that falls off when DNA is denatured. Specificity is guaranteed by amplicon-dependent Tm determined by melting curves.

3. CLINICAL DATA ON MELANOMA PATIENTS

3.1 Marker Genes

A number of genes encoding for melanosomal proteins are expressed specifically in melanocytes and melanomas. *Tyrosinase* is the first enzyme in the melanin biosynthesis pathway. It is a monooxygenase that catalyzes the conversion of tyrosine to dopa and of dopa to dopaquinone. *Tyrosinase* is, therefore, one of the most specific markers of melanocytes, and it is conserved in most amelanotic melanoma metastases. Expression of the *tyrosinase* gene is the most widely used indicator for the detection of circulating melanoma cells. Other melanocyte-specific proteins include gp100, which is recognized by the diagnostic antibodies HMB45 and NKI-beteb (10), Melan A/MART1 (11, 12) and a family of *tyrosinase*-related proteins. *gp100* is less suited for monitoring of melanoma, since it is known to be frequently lost during tumor progression (13, 14). The expression of *Melan-A/MART1* and *tyrosinase*-related proteins has been less well studied, but it has been shown that their expression is also lost in a significant percentage of metastatic lesions as detected by specific monoclonal antibodies (15, 16). Melanomas also express tumor-associated genes such as the MAGE family: about 60% of metastatic lesions are positive for *MAGE-1*, and 80% for *MAGE-3* as detected by PCR (17–20). The family of proteins encoded by these genes may, therefore, represent another useful marker for metastatic melanoma.

Smith *et al.* (21) reported in 1991 that circulating melanoma cells can be detected by PCR of *tyrosinase* mRNA. Their PCR assay is used most frequently today because of its optimal primer design. The primers, designated as HTYR1 to HTYR4, exploit the presence of two introns in the *tyrosinase* gene. HTYR1 spans an intron, and another intron is located between the nested primers HTYR3 and −4. This primer design virtually excludes amplification of genomic DNA.

The initial report led to a number of more detailed investigations on the presence of *tyrosinase* mRNA in the peripheral blood of melanoma patients (7, 9, 22–26). Non-melanoma controls were always negative for expression of *tyrosinase* using this technique, suggesting that normal melanocytes do not circulate in blood, and that the presence of *tyrosinase* mRNA can be considered to be an evidence for circulating melanoma cells.

3.2 Clinical Cross-sectional Analyses

The results reported for melanoma patients vary considerably between different laboratories (27) (Table 1 summarizes the results published until 2001). This is most obvious in Stage IV melanoma patients, where the percentage with evidence for circulating melanoma cells ranges between 0% and 100%. The most likely explanation for these discrepancies is methodological differences between laboratories. Sample processing affecting efficiency of RNA extraction and cDNA synthesis may play a major role. In particular, the use of Ficoll-Hypaq density-gradient separation prior to RNA extraction may significantly decrease the number of positive results in Stage IV patients. Quality-assurance initiatives have recently been undertaken (34) to assess and ultimately resolve the methodological differences, thus facilitating the comparison of results from different laboratories.

3.3 PCR Data and Clinical Course

3.3.1 Early Stages

The detection of circulating melanoma cells could be particularly useful in earlier stages of the disease, and could ultimately guide decisions concerning adjuvant treatment strategies. To date, however, the percentage of patients with Stage I, II, and III melanoma and the PCR evidence for circulating melanoma cells in these patients varies considerably from one report to the next. This may be not only due to differences in methodology, but also to differences in patient selection.

Several early analyses, however, have already suggested that PCR results are of prognostic value in melanoma: Battyani *et al.* (23) described, that after resection of regional lymph node metastases, the likelihood of recurrence within 4 months was significantly higher in patients with a positive *tyrosinase* signal using PCR, and that patients with Stage IV disease and a positive *tyrosinase* signal were significantly more likely to experience rapid disease progression within 4 months than patients tested negative in the PCR assay. Mellado *et al.* (28) reported, in a prospective investigation of Stage II and III melanoma, that the

Table 1. Twenty-nine studies summarized for *tyrosinase* RT-PCR positivity in blood samples of melanoma patients with different stages (#)

Study	Stage I/II	Stage III	Stage IV	Negative Controls
Smith *et al.*, 1991 (21)	0	0/1	4/6	0/8
Brossart *et al.*, 1993 (7)	1/10	6/17	29/29	0/56
Battyani *et al.*, 1995 (23)	2/10	8/18	16/32	0/14
Hoon *et al.*, 1995 (24)	13/17	31/36	63/66	0/39
Foss *et al.*, 1995 (25)	0	0	0/6	2/31
Kunter *et al.*, 1996 (26)	0/16	0/14	9/34	0/9
Mellado *et al.*, 1996 (28)	14/39	7/17	33/35	0/50
Stevens *et al.*, 1996 (35)	1/5	2/4	2/3	0/25
Glaser *et al.*, 1997 (36)	1/43	0/15	12/44	0/35
Reinhold *et al.*, 1997 (37)	0/31	1/21	5/13	0/20
Jung *et al.*, 1997 (38)	0	0	13/50	0/15
Tessier *et al.*, 1997 (39)	0/42	0/20†	16/23	0/20
Farthmann *et al.*, 1998 (40)	6/46	7/41	16/36	0/20
Ghossein *et al.*, 1998 (41)	2/16	6/40	1/17	0/25
O'Connell *et al.*, 1998 (42)	2/4	3/9	2/3	0/5
Voit *et al.*, 1999 (43)	2/28	11/24	9/12	0/15
Palmieri *et al.*, 1999 (44)	53/154	24/49	24/32	0/41
Mellado *et al.*, 1999 (45)	2/11	6/33	2/13	0/8
Le Bricon *et al.*, 1999 (46)	0	1/10	4/20	0/1
Schittek *et al.*, 1999 (47)	21/119	8/48	21/58	0/40
Curry *et al.*, 1999 (48)	34/89	55/97	0	0/50
Hanekom *et al.*, 1999 (49)	10/143	0/10	0/12	0/1
Alao *et al.*, 1999 (50)	0	1/4	5/17	0/12
Kopreski *et al.*, 1999 (51)	0	0	4/6	0/20
de Vries *et al.*, 1999 (52)	2/6	4/27	15/73	0/10
Proebstle *et al.*, 2000 (53)	22/162	8/26	16/24	0
Brownbridge *et al.*, 2001 (54)	94/177	70/85	30/37	0/52
Reinhold *et al.*, 2001 (55)	5/30	5/14	7/16	2/28(*)
Stoitchkov *et al.*, 2001 (56)	0	0/14	2/6	0/16
Total	287/1198	264/694	360/743	4/666

Notes

data are given as number of *tyrosinase*-positive patients/total number of patients in the particular stage. NS indicates not separated. Thirty-two high-risk post-nodal dissection patients were not included (58 samples, not patients, tested).

† Negative at initial testing with other specimens. Patients were retested with transient positivity.

(*) Collaborative study, two out of seven laboratories provided false positive results for the control panel.

presence of *tyrosinase* transcripts in the peripheral blood was associated with significantly shorter disease-free survival.

Larger prospective investigations are necessary, and are still under way, in the EORTC and also in the US (Sunbelt trial) to confirm the prognostic value of the PCR assay, especially in melanoma patients with disease Stages I through III who have been rendered disease-free by surgery. These studies will also address the value of adjuvant treatment strategies (e.g., interferon-α (IFN-α) in PCR positive and negative patients in the setting of large controlled clinical trials), and thereby investigate the possibility of guiding treatment decisions based on PCR results.

3.3.2 Stage IV

In melanoma patients with Stage IV disease who have entered long-term complete remission upon treatment with IFN-α and interleukin-2 (IL-2), with or without resection of residual metastases, *tyrosinase* transcripts could still be detected in most patients for a period of over 5 years without clinical evidence of recurrence. Semiquantitative assessment revealed a very low number of *tyrosinase* transcripts, equivalent to less than 100 SK mel 28 melanoma cells (29). It is not clarified whether a rise in signal intensity could be an early indicator for relapse. It has to be acknowledged, that the amount of *tyrosinase* transcripts does not allow calculation of the number of circulating tumor cells, since the expression of the marker genes has been shown to vary between tumors in different persons (30) and is also expected to vary in the tumor of the same individual. This is especially important, when testing patients undergoing vaccination with melanocyte differentiation proteins. This specific immunologic treatment may lead to a selection of tumor cells with reduced or absent expression of marker genes, as already shown on the protein level in histologic samples (31) obtained in lesions regressing after non-specific immunotherapy with IFN-α and IL-2.

3.3.3 Tissue Analysis

The value of PCR for examination of solid tissue has been investigated. Lymph node preparations from patients with Stages I or II melanoma were analyzed pathologically and by PCR in one series of experiments (32). Of 29 regional lymph node samples, 38% had pathological evidence for melanoma cells, whereas 66% including all pathologically positive nodes, were RT-PCR positive as assessed by detection of *tyrosinase* mRNA. The results of lymph node investigation are very encouraging, but larger studies are necessary to discern the clinical value of this procedure (3). It is important to strictly avoid contact with skin when processing tissue samples to avoid contamination of the samples with melanocytes. For peripheral blood samples, the risk of contamination with skin melanocytes is lower, and may be further reduced by discarding the first syringe of blood drawn after venipuncture and using a second syringe to draw the sample for the PCR assay.

4. CONCLUSION AND FUTURE PROSPECTS

Quantification of tumor transcripts amplified by real-time PCR is a powerful and, in principle, the most sensitive tool to monitor the course of disease, to evaluate the response to chemotherapy in more detail and to identify patients at high risk for developing hematogenous melanoma metastasis or relapse (33, 34). If residual tumor cells are detected and the transcript amount of their tumor marker is even quantitated, clinicians could theoretically intervene early with therapy.

Prior to widespread application of these methods, it is important to first establish very rigid quality assurance systems for academic centers and, in the future, for commercial laboratories. Second, detection of molecular signals of potential occult tumor cells by PCR cannot automatically be regarded as defining tumor cell presence and competence for further metastases, or a disease stage warranting systemic treatment. To establish clinical utility and to test the prognostic value of PCR results, large prospective studies with a long follow-up period are needed and have been initiated within the EORTC Melanoma Group and the US Sunbelt trial in association with state-of-the-art clinical and pathological evaluation.

REFERENCES

1. Caron M, Jorgensen G, Rigel D, Friedman R. In: Blach CM, Houghton AN, Miltron GM, editors. The Worldwide Incidence of Malignant Melanoma. Philadelphia: JB Lippincott, 1992, pp. 27–45.
2. Lakhani S, Selby P, Bliss JM, Perren TJ, Gore ME, McElwain TJ. Chemotherapy for malignant melanoma: combinations and high doses produce more responses without survival benefit. Brit J Cancer. 1990; 61: 330–334.
3. Buzaid AC and Balch CM. Polymerase chain reaction of melanoma in peripheral blood: too early to assess clinical value. J Natl Cancer Inst. 1996; 88: 569–570.
4. Cross NC, Feng L, Chase A *et al.* Competitive polymerase chain reaction to estimate the number of bcr-abl transcripts in chronic myeloid leukemia patients after bone marrow transplantation. Blood. 1993; 82: 1929–1936.
5. Fukuhara T, Hooper WC, Baylin SB *et al.* Use of the polymerase chain reaction to detect hypermethylation in the calcitonin gene – a new, sensitive approach to monitor tumor cells in acute myelogenous leukemia. Leukemia Res. 1992; 16: 1031–1040.
6. Curry BJ, Smith MJ, Hersey P. Detection and quantitation of melanoma cells in the circulation of patients. Melanoma Res. 1996; 6: 45–54.
7. Brossart P, Keilholz U, Willhauck M, Scheibenbogen C *et al.* Hematogenous spread of malignant melanoma cells in different stages of disease. J Invest Dermatol. 1993; 101: 887–889.
8. Brossart P, Schmier J-W, Krüger S *et al.* A polymerase chain reaction-based semiquantitative assessment of malignant melanoma cells in peripheral blood. Cancer Res. 1995; 55: 4056–4068.
9. Brossart P, Keilholz U, Scheibenbogen C *et al.* Detection of residual tumor cells in patients with malignant melanoma responding to immunotherapy. J Immunotherapy. 1994; 15: 38–41.
10. Adema G, de Boer AJ, van't Hullenaar R *et al.* Melanocyte lineage-specific antigens recognized by monoclonal antibodies NKI-beteb, HMB-50, and HMB-45 are encoded by a single cDNA. Am J Path. 1993; 143: 1579–1585.

11. Adema GJ, de Boer AJ, Vogel AM *et al.* Molecular characterization of the melanoma lineage-specific antigen gp100. J Biol Chem. 1994; 269: 20126–20133.
12. Kawakami Y, Eliyahu S, Delgado CH *et al.* Cloning the gene coding for a shared human melanoma antigen recognized by autologous T cells infiltrating into tumor. Proc Natl Acad Sci USA. 1994; 91: 3515–3519.
13. Carrel S, Dore JF, Ruiter D *et al.* The EORTC melanoma group exchange program: evaluation of a multicenter monoclonal antibody study. Int J Cancer. 1991; 48: 836–847.
14. Scheibenbogen C, Weyers I, Ruiter D, Willhauck M, Bittinger A, Keilholz U. Expression of gp100 in melanoma metastases resected before or after treatment with IFN alpha and IL-2. J Immunother 1996; 19: 375–380.
15. Chen YT, Stockert E, Tsang S *et al.* Immunophenotyping of melanomas for tyrosinase: implications for vaccine development. Proc Natl Acad Sci USA. 1995; 92: 8125–8129.
16. Marincola FM, HiJazi YM, Fetsch P *et al.* Analysis of expression of the melanoma-associated antigens MART-1 and gp100 in metastatic melanoma cell lines and in situ lesions. J Immunotherapy. 1996; 19: 192–205.
17. Coulie PG, Brichard V, van Pel A *et al.* A new gene coding for a differentiation antigen recognized by autologous cytoloytic T lymphocytes on HLA-A2 melanomas. J Exp Med. 1994; 180: 35–42.
18. Gaugler B, Van den Eynde B, van der Bruggen P *et al.* Human gene MAGE-3 codes for an antigen recognized on a melanoma by autologous cytoloytic T lymphocytes. J Exp Med. 1994; 179: 921–930.
19. Brasseur F, Rimoldi D, Lienard D *et al.* Expression of MAGE genes in primary and metastatic cutaneous melanoma. Int J Cancer. 1995; 63: 375–380.
20. De Plaen E, Arden K, Traversari C *et al.* Structure, chromosomal localization and expression of twelve genes of the MAGE family. Immunogenetics. 1994; 40: 360–369.
21. Smith B, Selby P, Southgate J *et al.* Detection of melanoma cells in peripheral blood by means of reverse transcriptase and polymerase chain reaction. Lancet. 1991; 338: 1227–1229.
22. Tobal K, Sherman LS, Foss AJ, Lightman SL. Detection of melanocytes from uveal melanoma in peripheral blood using the polymerase chain reaction. Invest Ophthalmol Vis Sci. 1993; 34: 2622–2625.
23. Battyani Z, Grob J, Xerri L *et al.* PCR detection of circulating melanocytes as a prognostic marker in patients with melanoma. Arch Dermatol. 1995; 131: 443–447.
24. Hoon DS, Wang Y, Dale PS *et al.* Detection of occult melanoma cells in blood with a multiple-marker polymerase chain reaction assay. J Clin Oncol. 1995; 13: 2109–2116.
25. Foss AJ, Guille MJ, Occleston NL *et al.* The detection of melanoma cells in peripheral blood by reverse transcription polymerase chain reaction. Brit J Cancer. 1995; 72: 155–159.
26. Kunter U, Buer J, Probst M *et al.* Peripheral blood tyrosinase messenger RNA detection and survival in malignant melanoma. J Natl Cancer Inst. 1996; 88: 590–594.
27. Tsao H, Nadiminti U, Sober AJ, Bigby M. A meta-analysis of reverse transcriptase-polymerase chain reaction for tyrosinase mRNA as a marker for circulating tumor cells in cutaneous melanoma. Arch Dermatol. 2001; 137: 325–330.
28. Mellado B, Colomer D, Castel T *et al.* Detection of circulating neoplastic cells by reverse-transcriptase polymerase chain reaction in malignant melanoma: association with clinical stage and prognosis. J Clin Oncol. 1996; 14: 2091–2097.

29. de Vries TJ, Fourkour A, Punt CJ, van de Locht LT *et al*. Reproducibility of detection of tyrosinase and MART-1 transcripts in the peripheral blood of melanoma patients: a quality control study using real-time quantitative RT-PCR. Brit J Cancer. 1999; 80: 883–891.
30. Chen YT, Stockert E, Tsang S *et al*. Immunophenotyping of melanomas for tyrosinase: implications for vaccine development. Proc Natl Acad Sci USA. 1995; 92: 8125–8129.
31. Scheibenbogen C, Weyers I, Ruiter D *et al*. Expression of gp100 in melanoma metastases resected before or after treatment with IFN alpha and IL-2. J Immunother Emphasis Tumor Immunol. 1996; 19: 375–380.
32. Wang X, Heller R, VanVoorhis N, Cruse CW *et al*. Detection of submicroscopic lymph node metastases with polymerase chain reaction in patients with malignant melanoma. Ann Surg. 1994; 220: 768–774.
33. Max N, Wolf K, Spike B *et al*. Nested quantitative real-time PCR for detection of occult tumor cells. Recent Results Cancer Res. 2001; 158: 25–31.
34. Keilholz U, Willhauck M, Rimoldi D, Brasseur F, Dummer W, Rass K, de Vries T, Blaheta J, Voit C, Lrthe B, Burchill L. Reliability of reverse transcription-polymerase chain reaction (RT-PCR)-based assays for the detection of circulating tumor cells: a quality-assurance initiative of the EORTC melanoma cooperative group. EJC. 1998; 34: 750–753.
35. Stevens GL, Scheer WD, Levine EA. Detection of tyrosinase mRNA from the blood of melanoma patients. Cancer Epidemiol Biomarkers Prev. 1996; 5: 293–296.
36. Glaser R, Rass K, Seiter S *et al*. Detection of circulating melanoma cells by specific amplification of tyrosinase complementary DNA is not a reliable tumor marker in melanoma patients: a clinical two-center study. J Clin Oncol. 1997; 15: 2818–2825.
37. Reinhold U, Ludtke-Handjery HC, Schnautz S *et al*. The analysis of tyrosinase-specific mRNA in blood samples of melanoma patients by RT-PCR is not a useful test for metastatic tumor progression. J Invest Dermatol. 1997; 108: 166–169.
38. Jung FA, Buzaid AC, Ross MI *et al*. Evaluation of tyrosinase mRNA as a tumor marker in the blood of melanoma patients. J Clin Oncol. 1997; 15: 2826–2831.
39. Tessier MH, Denis MG, Lustenberger P, Dreno B. Detection of circulating neoplastic cells by reverse transcriptase and polymerase chain reaction in melanoma. Ann Dermatol Verel. 1997; 124: 607–611.
40. Farthmann B, Eberle J, Krasagakis K *et al*. RT-PCR for tyrosinase-mRNA positive cells in peripheral blood: evaluation strategy and correlation with known prognostic markers in 123 melanoma patients. J Invest Dermatol. 1998; 110: 263–267.
41. Ghossein RA, Coit D, Brennan M *et al*. Prognostic significance of peripheral blood and bone marrow tyrosinase messenger RNA in malignant melanoma. Clin Cancer Res. 1998; 4: 419–428.
42. O'Connell CD, Juhasz A, Kuo C *et al*. Detection of tyrosinase mRNA in melanoma by reverse transcription PCR and electrochemiluminescence. Clin Chem. 1998; 44: 1161–1169.
43. Voit C, Schoengen A, Schwurzer M *et al*. Detection of regional melanoma metastases by ultrasound B-scan, cytology or tyrosinase RT-PCR of fine-needle aspirates. Brit J Cancer. 1999; 80: 1672–1677.
44. Palmieri G, Strazzullo M, Ascierto PA *et al*. Polymerase chain reaction-based detection of circulating melanoma cells as an effective marker of tumor progression. Melanoma Cooperative Group. J Clin Oncol. 1999; 17: 304–311.
45. Mellado B, Gutierrez L, Castel T *et al*. Prognostic siginificance of the detection of circulating malignant cells by reverse transcriptase polymerase chain reaction in

long-term clinically disease-free melanoma patients. Clin Cancer Res. 1999; 5: 1843–1848.
46. Le Bricon T, Stoitchkov K, Letellier S *et al.* Simultaneous analysis of tyrosinase mRNA and markers of tyrosinase activity in the blood of patients with metastatic melanoma. Clin Chim Acta. 1999; 282: 101–113.
47. Schittek B, Bodingbauer Y, Ellwanger U *et al.* Amplification of MelanA messenger RNA in addition to tyrosinase increases sensitivity of melanoma cell detection in peripheral blood and is associated with the clinical stage and prognosis of malignant melanoma. Brit J Dermatol. 1999; 141: 30–36.
48. Curry BJ, Myers K, Hersey P. MART-1 is expressed less frequently on circulating melanoma cells in patients who develop distant compared with locoregional metastases. J Clin Oncol. 1999; 17: 2562–2571.
49. Hanekom GS, Stubbings HM, Johnson CA, Kidson SH. The detection of circulating melanoma cells correlates with tumor thickness and ulceration but is not predictive of metastasis for patients with primary melanoma. Melanoma Res. 1999; 9: 465–473.
50. Alao JP, Mohammed MQ, Slade MJ, Retsas S. Detection of tyrosinase mRNA by RT-PCR in the peripheral blood of patients with advanced metastatic melanoma. Melanoma Res. 1999; 9: 395–399.
51. Kopreski MS, Benko FA, Kwak LW, Gocke CD. Detection of tumor messenger RNA in the serum of patients with malignant melanoma. Clin Cancer Res. 1999; 5: 1961–1965.
52. de Vries TJ, Fourkour A, Punt CJ, van de Locht LT, Wobbes T, van den Bosch S, de Rooij MJ, Mensink EJ, Ruiter DJ, van Muijen GN. Reproducibility of detection of tyrosinase and MART-1 transcripts in the peripheral blood of melanoma patients: a quality control study using real-time quantitative RT-PCR. Br J Cancer 1999; 80: 883–91.
53. Proebstle TM, Jiang W, Hogel J, Keilholz U, Weber L, Voit C. Correlation of positive RT-PCR for tyrosinase in peripheral blood of malignant melanoma patients with clinical stage, survival and other risk factors. Brit J Cancer. 2000; 82: 118–123.
54. Brownbridge GG, Gold J, Edward M, MacKie RM. Evaluation of the use of tyrosinase-specific and melanA/MART-1-specific reverse transcriptase-coupled-polymerase chain reaction to detect melanoma cells in peripheral blood samples from 299 patients with malignant melanoma. Br J Dermatol. 2001; 144: 279–287.
55. Reinhold U, Berkin C, Bosserhoff AK, Deutschmann A *et al.* Interlaboratory evaluation of a new reverse transcriptase polymerase chain reaction-based enzyme-linked immunosorbent assay for the detection of circulating melanoma cells: a multicenter study of the Dermatologic Cooperative Oncology Group. J Clin Oncol. 2001; 19: 1723–1727.
56. Stoitchkov K, Letellier S, Garnier JP, Toneva M, Naumova E, Peytcheva E, Tzankov N, Bousquet B, Morel P, Le Bricon T. Evaluation of standard tyrosinase RT-PCR in melanoma patients by the use of the LightCycler system. Clin Chim Acta. 2001; 306: 133–138.

INDEX